Care of Older Adults
A strengths-based approach

Care of Older Adults: A strengths-based approach is a comprehensive introduction to aged care for the nursing profession in clinical practice. By taking a strengths-based approach, the book encourages practice with a focus on individuals' potential and capacities rather than their limits. Theories of ageing are linked with the older individual's strengths to ensure the text is well framed from an evidence base, as well as a clinical orientation.

Divided into three parts, the book presents the topic from a healthy ageing perspective through to chronic illness, frailty and end of life. Each chapter includes discussion and reflective questions, and concludes with a list of key points summarising the central content. Case studies combine evidence-based knowledge with practical examples in a number of aged-care settings.

Written by internationally renowned authors with extensive practical experience in aged care, *Care of Older Adults* provides undergraduate students in Australia and New Zealand with local content and a nursing focus.

Care of Older Adults

Adults

A strengths-based approach

Wendy Moyle   *Deborah Parker*   *Marguerite Bramble*

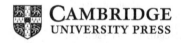

CAMBRIDGE
UNIVERSITY PRESS

CAMBRIDGE
UNIVERSITY PRESS

University Printing House, Cambridge CB2 8BS, United Kingdom

One Liberty Plaza, 20th Floor, New York, NY 10006, USA

477 Williamstown Road, Port Melbourne, VIC 3207, Australia

314-321, 3rd Floor, Plot 3, Splendor Forum, Jasola District Centre, New Delhi - 110025, India

79 Anson Road, #06-04/06, Singapore 079906

Cambridge University Press is part of the University of Cambridge.

It furthers the University's mission by disseminating knowledge in the pursuit of education, learning and research at the highest international levels of excellence.

www.cambridge.org
Information on this title: www.cambridge.org/9781107625457

First published 2014

Cover designed by Leigh Ashforth
Typeset by Aptara Corp.

A catalogue record for this publication is available from the British Library

A catalogue record for this publication is available from the British Library of the National Library of Australia at www.nla.gov.au

ISBN 978-1-107-62545-7 Paperback

....

Every effort has been made in preparing this book to provide accurate and up-to-date information which is in accord with accepted standards and practice at the time of publication. Although case histories are drawn from actual cases, every effort has been made to disguise the identities of the individuals involved. Nevertheless, the authors, editors and publishers can make no warranties that the information contained herein is totally free from error, not least because clinical standards are constantly changing through research and regulation. The authors, editors and publishers therefore disclaim all liability for direct or consequential damages resulting from the use of material contained in this book. Readers are strongly advised to pay careful attention to information provided by the manufacturer of any drugs or equipment that they plan to use.

Foreword

One of life's truisms is that we will all experience ageing. Most of us won't think about it until the effects of ageing give us either a gentle nudge or a hard wake-up call. Either way, when we are confronted with its effects, quite reasonably we won't want it to define us. Rather the effects and changes of ageing will be woven into the fabric of what makes us unique as individuals.

Unfortunately in the western world the term 'ageing' has evolved to have negative connotations in a way that devalues the worth of the individual's contributions – past, present and future. Yet we know that the older person can be resilient, informed about their health issues and actively engaged in the decisions about their health and care requirements. As a health professional, adopting a strengths-based perspective means we can support the person and their family, acknowledging their strengths and resources rather than focusing on problems, vulnerabilities and potential deficits.

Therefore a strengths-based approach provides a context for practice and care that is positive, inclusive and empowering because it encourages the older adult to take control of their own life in meaningful and sustainable ways. Notably a strengths-based approach doesn't deny that a person experiences problems but rather takes account of these while attempting to identify the positive basis of the person's resources and strengths that will inform how they deal with the challenges resulting from the problems. A strengths-based approach to care offers a different language to describe the older adult's situation and enables health professionals to see opportunities and solutions, not merely problems. Identifying, acknowledging and working with strengths as a starting point for care is not the norm in health care services despite the obvious benefits of doing so.

The authors, Wendy Moyle, Deborah Parker and Marguerite Bramble, have given us a text that is informative, logically sequenced and easy to use as a reference to inform practice while challenging our current models of care delivery for older adults. They do this by embedding in each chapter principles that are not merely theoretical but that challenge us to also consider our values and attitudes, which we know shape the way we care for others. This text provides us with the knowledge we need to ensure our practice is about working in partnership with the older person and facilitating rather than always fixing, focusing on health/well-being within the context of their current health status rather than being constantly concerned with and belabouring deficits.

I congratulate the authors on their collaborative efforts to bring this excellent piece of work to fruition and believe this text can assist all health professionals providing care to the older person from the novice undergraduate, as they learn their profession, to the most advanced practitioner.

Professor Helen McCutcheon
Dean, Florence Nightingale School of Nursing and Midwifery
King's College, London

Contents

3   Principles of strengths-based care and other nursing models 33

Wendy Moyle

**4   Nursing older people across aged care settings:
     interdisciplinary and intradisciplinary approaches   49**

Marguerite Bramble

**5   Evidence-based nursing interventions in primary care:
     a strengths-based approach   67**

Marguerite Bramble

**12   A strengths-based palliative approach for the frail older
adult living in residential aged care   179**

Deborah Parker

**13   Evidence-based nursing interventions: a good death
and fostering pain relief   192**

Deborah Parker

About the authors

Wendy Moyle

PhD, MHSc, BN, Dip App Sci, RN

Wendy is the Director of the Centre for Health Practice Innovation (HPI), a research program in the Griffith Health Institute at Griffith University, Brisbane, Queensland. She is also a research leader in a National Dementia Collaborative Research Centre – Consumers and Carers and the Dementia Training and Study Centre at QUT. Her research focus has been on finding evidence for managing behavioural and psychological symptoms of dementia using controlled trials to test psychosocial interventions, assistive technologies, social robots, and complementary and alternative medicine interventions.

Deborah Parker

PhD, MSocSc, BA, Grad Cert Gerontology, Grad Cert Executive Leadership, RN

Deborah is the Director of the University of Queensland/Blue Care Research and Practice Development Centre and the Australian Centre for Evidence Based Community Care based at the University of Queensland, Brisbane, Queensland. Her research focus is on palliative aged care, dementia and evaluation of health services for older people.

Marguerite Bramble

PhD, BN (Hons), BEc, Grad Cert Research Mgmt, Grad Cert Strat Marketing, RN

Marguerite is a nurse academic with a passion for improving clinical practice, education and research in aged care. Currently Marguerite is Project Manager for a National Health and Medical Research Council (NHMRC) funded project in the Centre for Health Practice Innovation (HPI), a research program in the Griffith Health Institute at Griffith University, Brisbane, Queensland. She is also an adjunct senior lecturer with the University of Tasmania, where her teaching and supervisory focus is aged care and dementia care. Marguerite's research has involved a partnership intervention for family caregivers of people with dementia.

Acknowledgements

For my husband Rob, who has travelled the journey with me, and my parents who provided excellent role models of successful ageing.

Wendy Moyle

For my husband Mike, whose support never wavers and my father Joe, who as one of the old-old continues to provide a constant source for me to reflect on ageing and senescence.

Marguerite Bramble

Part 1

Ageing and gerontology

1 What is ageing?

Marguerite Bramble

Learning objectives

After reading this chapter you will be able to:

1   Define ageing in the context of caring for older adults.

2   Outline how the multidimensional theories of ageing link to the characteristics of old age.

3   Explain how the science of gerontology builds a body of knowledge and competence in gerontological nursing.

4   Describe future trends in ageing and gerontological nursing.

Introduction

In developing a personal and professional **philosophy** of ageing, we essentially build on our personal experience and this is common to all of us. For nurses in practice reflecting on the ageing experience and developing the capability to care for older people in the context of the human **lifespan** is instrumental to providing holistic, person-centred care. **Holistic care** is described as a system of comprehensive patient care that considers the multidimensional physical, emotional, social, economic and spiritual needs of the person; his or her response to illness; and the effect of the illness on the ability to meet self-care needs. **Person-centred care** is described as the treatment and care provided by health services that places the person at the centre of their own care and considers the needs of the older person's carers (C. Brown, 2010).

The International Council of Nurses (2010) addresses these concepts by describing the discipline of nursing as follows:

> Nursing encompasses autonomous and collaborative care of individuals of all ages, families, groups and communities, sick or well and in all settings. Nursing includes the promotion of health, prevention of illness, and the care of ill, disabled and dying people.

Philosophy The values and beliefs of a discipline.

Lifespan The period between birth and death.

Holistic care A system of comprehensive patient care that considers the physical, emotional, social, economic and spiritual needs of the person; his or her response to illness; and the effect of the illness on the ability to meet self-care needs.

Person-centred care Treatment and care provided by health services that places the person at the centre of their own care and considers the needs of the older person's carers.

In Australia, although the development of specialised care of older people, termed 'gerontological nursing', has been relatively recent, **gerontology** knowledge and models of care are drawn from international core nursing values and principles, including health promotion and protection, prevention and treatment of disease, and improving quality of care within current clinical practice guidelines (Tabloski, 2010).

Gerontology
The study of ageing.

The scope of gerontological nursing involves using comprehensive **geriatric** evaluation to fully understand the needs of the older person, particularly when transitioning between clinical contexts such as acute, subacute, rehabilitation, community and residential care (Tabloski, 2010). This comprehensive evaluation is multidimensional and involves professionals from other disciplines such as geriatricians and psychiatrists, social workers, psychologists, physiotherapists and occupational therapists. The focus for nurses is on assessing functional capacity in the physical, social and psychological domains (Tabloski, 2010). The multidimensional approach to the provision of care will be examined further in Chapter 2.

Geriatric
The clinical practice of medicine that encompasses the gerontology, pathology and complexities of ageing.

Whilst theoretical frameworks and models of care will be presented that relate to contemporary nursing practice, the overarching framework used within this textbook is strengths-based nursing. This framework is described in detail in Chapter 3. Where relevant, reference to the professional codes of conduct developed by the Australian Nursing and Midwifery Council and Nursing Council of New Zealand will also be made.

What is ageing?

Ageing is very simply described as the process of growing old and occurs universally as a natural part of all life and experience of living. For human beings ageing is described as a multidimensional process and is viewed from both the subjective or humanistic, and objective or scientific perspectives, beginning at birth (Hunter, 2012). As human life expectancy and the human lifespan continue to increase in the 21st century, nursing care will involve a higher proportion of older people, making it increasingly important for nurses to understand the multidimensional impacts of ageing and how we define 'old age' (Australian Institute of Health and Welfare, 2007). This multidimensional approach includes all aspects of how people age from chronological, biological, physiological, biomedical, psychological, social, cultural, spiritual and economic perspectives.

Chronological age

Chronological age is defined as the length of time that has passed since birth (Hunter, 2012). Since the beginning of the 20th century chronologically 65 years and older continues to be a measurement of being 'old' (P. Brown, 2010; Staab & Hodges, 1996). However, there have been a number of significant changes during the last century that have resulted in the need for us to rethink this socially determined notion of 'old age'. Generalisations about all people who are 65 years and older are likely to be an inaccurate indicator of a person's well-being, physical fitness and mental capability (Butler, Lewis & Sunderland, 1998; Moschis, 1996). Firstly, the average length of time human beings can expect to live, or **life expectancy**, has increased as a result of fewer deaths in childhood and early adulthood, improved drugs and medical technology, and better disease prevention (Touhy & Jett, 2012). Secondly, as a result of both humanistic and scientific research we have a greater understanding of the **human lifespan**, or how long the human species can potentially live, with current estimations at around 116 years (Fillit, Rockwood & Woodhouse, 2010; Hunter, 2012). Many factors, however, interact to ensure that most people die well short of this theoretical maximum limit, including genetic traits and disorders, behaviour and lifestyle, environmental and social settings, accidents and injuries, infections, coexisting conditions, social support, disease management, and health care quality and accessibility (Anstey et al., 2010).

Life expectancy
The number of years that an individual is expected to live as determined by statistics.

Human lifespan
How long a member of the human species can potentially live.

In summary, whilst the dramatic change in chronological life expectancy has fuelled the examination of human ageing from a lifespan (or death) end point, this does not take into account the complexities of the experience for each individual as they age, or the tensions for nurses and health professionals between maximising an individual's lifespan versus that person's **quality of life** (Fillit et al., 2010).

Quality of life
An individual's perception of their position in life in the context of the culture and value systems in which they live and in relation to their goals, expectations, standards and concerns.

Biological and physiological ageing

In recent times our knowledge about human biological ageing has developed as a result of describing and cataloguing ageing changes at a cellular level in more short-lived species such as nematodes, fruit flies and mice (Fillit et al., 2010).

Scientists describe biological ageing from a biological perspective as an exceedingly complex process of physiological change (Hunter, 2012). Scientists now know that once people have reached and passed maturity in their 20s and early 30s there is an increasing likelihood that these physiological ageing changes may become detrimental to health. The transition from maturity to this next life stage of physiological ageing is known as **senescence** (Fillit et al., 2010).

Senescence
Physiological progressive deterioration of body systems that can increase mortality risk in an older person.

The physiological ageing changes or degree of senescence experienced by each person's body system associated with ageing differs for each individual across the human lifespan. It is important for nurses to understand that physiological changes and ageing are not simply associated with deterioration. For many older people the normal changes associated with ageing may be described as beneficial or neutral (Fillit et al., 2010; Tabloski, 2010). However, as a person ages, they are increasingly at risk of injury, illness and death (Fillit et al., 2010). These risks are further discussed in Chapter 2, p. 19 and p. 24.

In the context of normal physiological changes of ageing it is important for nurses in practice to understand that chronological age is just one major **risk factor** for development of most age-related pathologies or illnesses. It is also important to understand that, physiologically, human maturity and ageing starts during young adulthood, and premature ageing may be caused by many damaging but modifiable influences, such as smoking, diet and exercise (Tabloski, 2010). One way to distinguish chronological age from physiological age is to understand the normal changes of ageing. In practice older clients will have some evidence of normal physiological changes of ageing, as described in Table 1.1. However it is important to remember that increasing chronological age is just one of the major risk factors for development of most age-related pathologies or illnesses.

Risk factor(s)
Behaviour(s) that increase risk of disease.

Multidimensional ageing frameworks and theories

As discussed in the previous section, from both scientific and humanistic perspectives it is almost impossible to understand the complexities of ageing by simply linking the physiological changes of ageing to a person's chronological age. In order to assist our understanding of these complexities we will examine the development of ageing frameworks and theories within the sociological, nursing, medical and psychological disciplines.

TABLE 1.1 *Normal physiological changes of ageing*

ORGAN OR ORGAN SYSTEM AFFECTED	AGEING CHANGES
Heart	Heart muscle thickens affecting maximum pumping rate and body's ability to extract oxygen from blood.
Arteries	Arteries become less elastic. The older heart beats harder to supply energy to propel blood forward.
Lungs	Maximum breathing capacity may decline by about 40% between the ages of 40 and 70 years.
Brain	Brain loses some of the axons and neurons that connect with each other.
Kidneys	Kidneys gradually become less efficient at removing waste from the body.
Bladder	Bladder capacity declines.
Body fat	Weight tends to decline due to loss of muscle and fat. Fat is redistributed to deeper organs from skin, increasing vulnerability to heart disease.
Muscles	Without exercise muscle mass declines from age 40 to age 70. Exercise can slow this rate of loss.
Bones	Bone mineral is lost throughout life. Loss outpaces replacement for women at about age 35 and is accelerated at menopause.
Sight	Deterioration begins in the 40s. At age 70 ability to distinguish fine details begins to decline.
Hearing	With middle age it becomes more difficult to hear higher frequencies. Older adults may have difficulty distinguishing vowels and understanding speech. Hearing deteriorates more quickly in men than women.
Personality	Personality usually does not change radically, however older people who experience health problems, chronic illness and pain are at risk from depression and social isolation.

Source: Adapted from Tabloski, 2010, p. 18

The development of sociology and ageing

The discipline of sociology arose as a mode of knowledge concerned with the moral problems of modern society. In the context of ageing it focuses on the social and environmental realities of older persons (Butler et al., 1998).

> **Ageism** A set of beliefs, attitudes, norms and values used to justify age-based prejudice and discrimination.

With the increase in older persons in society comes the issue of implicit **ageism**, in which ageing stereotypes are unconsciously triggered and associated with social isolation, physical and mental burden, and death (Hunter, 2012; Levy, 2001; Minichiello, Browne & Kendig, 2000). Models of healthy ageing have been developed to counteract this 'ageing anxiety' and to clarify myths about age-related psychosocial and functional changes (Hunter, 2012). Such models that emphasise optimising physical, mental and social well-being and function have provided the framework for social and economic government policies including 'Healthy Ageing' and 'Successful Ageing'. However it is argued that these policies tend to promote societal values based on lifestyle and consumption choices with very little reflection on ethical and cultural considerations integral to providing comprehensive nursing care for adults in practice (Cardona, 2008).

From a sociological perspective, therefore, socially constructed moral categories may create a tension for nurses in practice between traditional values associated with older people such as wisdom and disengagement and modern negative constructions of old age such as inactivity and dependence (Butler et al., 1998; Katz, 2002).

Theories of ageing

In general it is **theory** development that provides new approaches to developing nurses' understanding of complex phenomena such as ageing, and to identifying frameworks for the development of new models of nursing practice (Meleis, 1991; Touhy & Jett, 2012). As with the sociological context it must be remembered that no ageing theory on its own can address the individual experience of ageing. Similarly biomedical theories alone may reduce a person to a biomedical entity, ignoring both individual variation and the multiplicity of factors that go into making a person.

Theory The search for an explanation.

Sociological theories provide a moral and ethical framework for person-centred care, which focuses on the strengths and uniqueness of the individual, on maintaining their dignity and self-esteem, particularly those with cognitive decline (C. Brown, 2010). This philosophy of care, based on the Kantian notion of personhood, forms the basis for the core ethical principles that guide nursing practice and decision making and the competency framework for professional practice (C. Brown, 2010). The role of this textbook is to move the notion of person-centred care forward and to concentrate on a strengths-based model of care as a way of promoting the older person's strengths and overcoming the notion of deficits being identified in relation to ageing.

The biological, biomedical and psychological theories of ageing are important for the nursing profession as they provide a foundation for planning best practice transitional care and interventions, and accentuating the influence of culture, family, education, roles, patterns of disease and community (Staab & Hodges, 1996).

Psychosocial theories of ageing, such as role theory, continuity theory and Maslow's hierarchy of needs, attempt to describe changes in roles and relationships in later life and provide an important backdrop for understanding late life development and the notion of self-actualisation (Touhy & Jett, 2012). In contemporary practice notions such as 'gerotranscendence', derived from Jungian theory and empirical observation, offer opportunities for nurses to identify ways in which older people can develop beyond the expectations we have of them across the lifespan, and to higher levels of acceptance of self (Touhy & Jett, 2012). This spiritual dimension takes us beyond ideas of development based on sociological ideas of 'success' that are often applied to the 'middle-aged' and the 'younger-old' and links to the process of transition into the more expanded concept of senescence (Wadensten, 2007). The implications of these psychosocial theories of ageing will be discussed in Chapters 7 and 9.

Ageing theories and cultural considerations

Ageing theories and the western concept of the human lifespan and life cycle are very different from those of other cultures, such as indigenous cultures in Australia and New Zealand, and have a profound impact on how life and the concept of 'self' is experienced (Butler et al., 1998). Added to this is society's increasing secularisation of religious and spiritual values, which produces a void around the subject of death itself, resulting in its denial and the forming of cultural differences and barriers around older people (Butler et al., 1998). These differences can also add to the language and cultural barriers for older people from non-English speaking countries despite evidence that they are in better health generally and have a higher life expectancy (Australian Institute of Health and Welfare, 2007).

In summary, ageing theories that address the multiple processes of ageing continue to provide new insights to the nursing body of knowledge in gerontology. The development of evidence-based models of care from a transitional approach to ageing attempts to explain the why and the how through **interdisciplinary** ageing theories (Bengtson et al., 2009). In nursing we are poised to articulate gerontological knowledge with clinical practice to provide best practice holistic frameworks for care. Relevant ageing theories are summarised in Table 1.2.

Interdisciplinary
Involving the scope of two or more distinct disciplines.

TABLE 1.2 *Ageing theories relevant to nursing practice*

AGEING THEORY	DESCRIPTION	FRAMEWORK
Biological ageing theories	Endocrine Theory – Biological clock acts through hormones to control pace of ageing.	Biomedicine
	Immunological Theory – Programmed decline in immune systems leads to higher risk of illness.	Pathology
	Wear and Tear Theory – Abuse or neglect of an organ or body system can stimulate premature ageing and disease.	Biomedicine
	Free Radical Theory – Accumulated damage from oxygen radicals causes cells and organs to lose function and organ reserve.	Biomedicine; pharmacy
	Cross-link Theory – Binding between glucose and protein causes malfunction of protein, resulting in ageing.	Biomedicine; nutrition
	Somatic DNA Damage Theory – Genetic mutations accumulate with increasing age causing cells to malfunction.	Biomedicine; genetics
Psychological ageing theories	Theory of Individualism – Shift from the external world (extroversion) towards the inner experience (introversion).	Jungian Theory (1960)
	Developmental Theory – Stage of life where the individual faces ego integrity versus despair.	Erikson's Eight Stages of Life (1966)
Sociological ageing theories	Disengagement Theory – Older person and society engage in mutual withdrawal.	Cummings and Henry (1961)
	Activity Theory – Older adults should stay active and engaged to age successfully.	Havighurst, Neugarten & Tobin (1963)
Psychosocial Theories	Person–Environment Fit Theory – Changes and changing environments associated with ageing are a source of stress and affect well-being.	Powell Lawton (1975)
	Role Theory – As one ages the changing roles from social and environmental influences cause role stress and role conflict.	Biddle & Thomas (1966)
	Theory of Gerotranscendence – Human ageing, when optimised, leads to a new and qualitatively different perspective on life.	Wadenstein (2007)

The development of gerontology

As a discipline gerontology is defined as the scientific study of the effects of time on human development, specifically the study of older persons (Touhy &

Jett, 2012). Gerontology first emerged through medicine and the specialisation of geriatricians and then old age psychiatrists.

The discipline of gerontology was formed in the 1960s, spurning the instigation of early longitudinal studies focusing on older adults. Since then life expectancies have increased substantially and the early studies, whilst ground breaking, often did not contain many participants who lived past 85 years of age. Therefore, there is an increasing need for information on ageing of adults aged 80 years and older. Moreover, there is a great need for an understanding of individual ageing as a developmental process occurring over time, contextualised in socio-political, environmental and historical contexts (Anstey et al., 2011).

Gerontology involves all aspects of the person's life and encompasses the demographics of ageing, the biology of ageing, the neuropsychology of ageing and medical gerontology (Fillit et al., 2010; Tabloski, 2010). Through multiple theory development and research, gerontology continues to evolve as a **multidisciplinary** and interdisciplinary field involving biomedical, social, psychological, pathological and nursing disciplines (Fillit et al., 2010).

In acknowledgement of the importance of understanding 'senescence', biomedicine, or the interdisciplinary branch of medical **science** that applies biological and physiological principles to clinical practice, combines these disciplines to research disease pathologies specific to the ever-growing number of older people throughout the world. Hence the transitional approach commonly used in paediatrics as children develop to adulthood is increasingly used in the development of care programs for people over 65 years as they transition through senescence and the complexity of their needs increases.

Multidisciplinary Combining or involving several academic disciplines or professional specialisations in an approach to a topic or problem.

Science A unified body of knowledge about phenomena that is based on agreed-upon evidence.

The development of psychological life stages

The discipline of psychology is simply defined as the understanding of human behaviour and embraces all aspects of the human experience from child development to care for older people. From a psychological perspective, therefore, the human process of ageing has been artificially divided into stages and includes antepartum, neonate, toddler, child, adolescent, young adult, middle age and adult (Tabloski, 2010). As average life expectancy increases the psychology of human development has been expanded to include the entire lifespan and old age now includes the 'developmental stages' of the young-old (65–74), middle-old (75–84) and old-old (85 years and over) (Butler et al., 1998; Tabloski, 2010).

Currently psychologists, together with sociologists and physiologists, are taking an interdisciplinary approach to proposing differing models that describe successful adaptation to the long and unstable period of extreme old age, or the old-old, based on new frameworks that emphasise psychological development in old age and age-related differences in functional status (Gondo, 2012). These stages will be further discussed in Chapter 2.

The development of gerontological nursing

In Australia, no competency standards for gerontological nurses currently exist. Countries such as Canada have well-established gerontological nursing standards of practice and scope of practice with specialty career paths for gerontological nurses as practitioners, managers and educators (Canadian Gerontological Nursing Association (CGNA), 2010; Tabloski, 2010). Standards identified by the CGNA (2010) that will be addressed in this textbook are as follows:

> Gerontological nurses demonstrate leadership, and direct their attention toward promotion, prevention, maintenance, rehabilitation and the palliation of health related issues to address the functional needs, abilities, and expectations of older people and their family members. Gerontological nurses practice in a manner that incorporates normal age related changes in a socially constructed and culturally sensitive manner.

The gerontological nurse's role is to identify and utilise the functional strengths of the older person, to assist them to maximise their independence, minimise impacts of disability and disease, and where possible achieve a peaceful death (Tabloski, 2010). The overarching aim is to achieve a balance between the psychosocial, physical, cultural and spiritual needs of older people, between caring and a critical evaluation of the structures in which nurses are expected to care (Chenoworth, 2010; Dunlop, 1994). The scope of gerontological nursing has become more defined through the processes of continuous learning and of integrating research evidence and professional experience to guide practice (Chenoworth, 2010; Fillit et al., 2010).

Nursing curriculum should draw on multidisciplinary perspectives to develop the profession's body of knowledge with the aim to evaluate, monitor and protect an older person's functioning and quality of life, taking into account physiological, psychological, social and economic influences (P. Brown, 2010; Touhy & Jett, 2012). As the nursing discipline develops, new understandings of a person's transition to senescence, relying on simple medical diagnosis, assumes less importance and evaluation of the person's level of functioning and well-being takes on more significance (P. Brown, 2010). The interdisciplinary approach has seen the development of **functional assessment** tools and psychosocial measurements of quality of life, such as stress and well-being, that will be discussed in Chapters 3 and 5 (Touhy & Jett, 2012).

Functional assessment
Comprehensive evaluation of physical and cognitive abilities required to maintain independence.

Every older person should expect care provided by nurses with competence in gerontological nursing (Touhy & Jett, 2012). Ethical considerations and the nurses' ethical code of conduct shapes their ability to be there at the juncture of life's transitions, to provide support for individual health care and to reduce risks of increasing illness (Thomasa, 1994). Thus gerontological nursing involves both clinical and non-clinical capability and understanding that a 90 year old will most likely require different care from a 70 year old, just as care of a new born is different from a 16 year old (Touhy & Jett, 2012). The gerontological nurse must have the skills to evaluate and monitor the individual's journey from health to illness from a functional perspective, then to analyse what is going well, not just what is going wrong (Butler et al., 1998; Tabloski, 2010).

The future of ageing for nurses

The future of ageing practice in Australia and New Zealand will see nurse managers, clinicians and practitioners who utilise interdisciplinary and **intradisciplinary** clinical frameworks, and holistic rather than simple biomedical models that demonstrate use of nursing theory in practice (Chenitz, Stone & Salisbury, 1991; Staab & Hodges, 1996). As our understanding of ageing increases nurses will organise knowledge and problem solving around the effectiveness of evidence-based nursing interventions demonstrated in measurable outcomes

Intradisciplinary
Occurring within the scope of a discipline, between people active in the discipline.

(Chenoworth, 2010). Nursing research will continue to develop interdisciplinary theories as a framework for understanding the developmental processes of ageing and the transition into 'old age', and to develop capability models of care transitioning to palliative models based on individual needs (Tornstam, 2005). Further research will also continue to provide continuous improvement frameworks for screening, monitoring and assessment with the view to communicating the data to other nurses and health professionals in the multidisciplinary team and to the client (Brown, 2007; Tolson, Booth & Schofield, 2011).

As the discipline of gerontology becomes more formalised, Australian and New Zealand nurses working in the specialty will, as part of multidisciplinary research teams, interpret, apply and evaluate research findings to improve and inform nursing practice and capability (Tabloski, 2010). Specific competencies for gerontological nurses should be developed and adopted so that the direction and evaluation of this specialisation can be assured. In-depth discussion of multidisciplinary gerontological research will be further discussed in Chapter 2.

Personal and professional philosophy of ageing

Case scenario 1.1

You have recently graduated from university as a registered nurse. Your first clinical placement is in a subacute rehabilitation unit in a large metropolitan hospital. During a morning shift Jim, who is 78 years old, of Italian origin and comes from a family of market gardeners, becomes agitated about his inability to walk unassisted following a fall in his garden 10 days ago leading to a repair of his fractured hip. He is aggressive when you approach him about attending his mobility program, and refuses to eat or take his medications, saying they 'don't do anything for me'. Jim was diagnosed with osteoarthritis five years ago and at times has difficulties with constipation and a reduced appetite. He describes himself as 'full of aches and pains', 'ready for the scrap heap' and his future as 'grim' as he can no longer tend to his beloved garden or provide in this way for his extended family. When Jim's wife and two sons arrive with his favourite food they become distressed by Jim's actions, saying they 'just want him to be his old self' and 'to maintain his important role as a well respected older person in their large family and social network'. Jim's sons, who have started to adapt the garden to accommodate his changing abilities, approach you about his deteriorating situation.

You note from the morning's handover that Jim is described as struggling with his functional capacities and becoming very emotional. You explore his psychosocial history and geriatric assessment with your clinical mentor.

Reflective questions

Read and reflect on this case scenario and address the following questions:

> In developing a personal and professional philosophy of ageing, critically reflect on your most frequently held assumptions about how people age.

> As a registered nurse what do you see as the main ethical and cultural considerations in relation to Jim's situation? How does this relate to a holistic approach to care?

> In the context of theories of ageing presented in this chapter what are two perspectives presented by Jim and his family? What is the nurse's role in this situation?

> What do you feel is an appropriate response to Jim and his family?

> Explore the clinical mentor's role in supporting you as a new graduate in negotiating these processes.

Reflective activity

Consider case scenario 1.1 in relation to your nursing education and practice and think about the following:

- How were theories of ageing presented to you in your nursing education? Has this influenced your practice?
- Do you see examples of holistic assessment or geriatric assessment in practice?
- If so how would these assessment tools guide your practice when evaluating an individual's journey to senescence?

Summary

- Human ageing is a multidimensional process encompassing chronological, biological, physiological, biomedical, psychological, social, cultural, spiritual and economic perspectives.
- As human life expectancy and the lifespan increases, ageing theories inform nursing practice.
- The science of gerontology provides new knowledge to inform gerontological nursing practice.
- Gerontological nurses will work as part of multidisciplinary research teams to improve and inform nursing practice and capability.

Conclusion

This chapter aims to increase understanding and ability to reflect on the notion of ageing and the transition to old age as a natural part of life. The chapter began by defining chronological age in the context of normal physiological changes and senescence. Relevant frameworks and theories were presented as a basis for understanding the multiple processes of ageing and its normal, developmental impacts on the person. An overview of gerontology provides links to the scope of geronotological nursing practice and the future of ageing for nurses. This future involves using a holistic approach to support gerontological nurses in developing skills to evaluate and monitor each client's journey to senescence.

Further reading

You may also like to read the following websites, which provide information about ageing and life expectancy in Australia and New Zealand:

- Australian Government Department of Health – National Strategy for an Ageing Australia: http://www.health.gov.au/
- Australian Institute of Health and Welfare – publications related to ageing and health expectancy: http://www.aihw.gov.au/
- New Zealand Ministry of Social Development – The New Zealand Positive Ageing Strategy and Longer and Healthier Lives: http://www.msd.govt.nz/

References

Anstey, K., Birrell, C., Browning, C., Burns, R., Byles, J., Kiely, K., ... Ross, L. (2011). Understanding ageing in older Australians: The contribution of the Dynamic Analyses to Optimise Ageing (DYNOPTA) project to the evidence base and policy. *Australasian Journal on Ageing*, 30 (October), 24–31.

Anstey, K., Byles, J., Luszcz, M., Mitchell, P. Steel, D., Booth, H., ... Kendig, H. (2010). Cohort profile: The Dynamic Analyses to Optimize Ageing (DYNOPTA) project. *International Journal of Epidemiology*, 39(1), 44–51.

Australian Institute of Health and Welfare. (2007). *Older Australians at a Glance*. (4th edition). Canberra.

Bengtson, V., Silverstein, M., Putney, N. & Gans, D. (2009). *Handbook of Theories of Aging*. New York: Springer Publishing Company.

Brown, C. (2010). Person-centred care in aged care. In P. Brown (Ed.), *Health Care of the Older Adult: An Australian and New Zealand Nursing Perspective*. Warriewood, NSW: Woodslane Press.

Brown, P. (2010). Ageing and care of the older adult. In P. Brown (Ed.), *Health Care of the Older Adult: An Australian and New Zealand Nursing Perspective*. Warriewood, NSW: Woodslane Press Pty Ltd.

Brown, S. (2007). *Health and Illness in Older Adults*. Frenchs Forest: Pearson Education Australia.

Butler, R., Lewis, M. & Sunderland, T. (1998). *Aging and Mental Health*. Austin: PRO-ED.

Canadian Gerontological Nursing Association. (2010). *Gerontological Nursing Competencies and Standards of Practice 2010*. Vancouver.

Cardona, B. (2008). 'Healthy Ageing' policies and anti-ageing ideologies and practices: On the exercise of responsibility. *Medical Health Care and Philosophy*, 11, 475–83.

Chenitz, W., Stone, J. & Salisbury, S. (1991). *Clinical Gerontological Nursing*. Philadephia: W.B. Saunders Company.

Chenoworth, L. (2010). Evidence-based nursing practice. In P. Brown (Ed.), *Health Care of the Older Adult: An Australian and New Zealand Nursing Perspective*. Warriewood, NSW: Woodslane Press Pty Ltd.

Dunlop, M. (1994). Is a science of caring possible? In P. Benner (Ed.), *Interpretive Phenomenology: Embodiment, Caring and Ethics in Health and Illness*. Thousand Oaks: Sage Publications.

Fillit, H., Rockwood, K. & Woodhouse, K. (2010). *Textbook of Geriatric Medicine and Gerontology*. Philadelphia: Elsevier.

Gondo, Y. (2012). Longevity and successful ageing: Implications from the oldest old and centenarians. *Asian Journal of Gerontology & Geriatrics*, 7, 39–43.

Hunter, S. (2012). *Miller's Nursing for Wellness in Older Adults*. Philadelphia: Wolters Kluwer/Lippincott Williams & Wilkins.

International Council of Nurses. (2010). Definition of nursing [Website definition]. Retrieved from www.icn.ch/definition.htm

Katz, S. (2002). Growing older without aging? Positive aging, anti-ageism and anti-aging. *Generations*, 25(4), 27–32.

Levy, B. (2001). Eradication of ageism requires addressing the enemy within. *The Gerontologist*, 41, 578–9.

Meleis, A. (1991). *Theoretical Nursing: Development and Progress*. Philadelphia: J.B. Lippincott.

Minichiello, V., Browne, J. & Kendig, H. (2000). Perceptions and consequences of ageism: Views of older people. *Ageing and Society*, 20, 253–78.

Moschis, G. (1996). *Gerontographics; Life-stage Segmentation for Marketing Strategy Development*. Westport: Greenwood.

Staab, A. & Hodges, L. (1996). *Essentials of Gerontological Nursing: Adaptation to the Aging Process*. Philadelphia: J.B. Lippincott.

Tabloski, P. (2010). *Gerontological Nursing*. (2nd edition). New Jersey: Pearson.

Thomasa, D. (1994). Toward a new medical ethics. In P. Benner (Ed.), *Interpretive Phenomenology: Embodiment, Caring and Ethics in Health and Illness*. Thousand Oaks: Sage Publications.

Tolson, D., Booth, J. & Schofield, I. (2011). Principles of gerontological nursing. In D. Tolson, J. Booth & I. Schofield (Eds.), *Evidence Informed Nursing with Older People*. Oxford: Wiley-Blackwell.

Tornstam, L. (2005). *Gerotranscendence: A Developmental Theory of Positive Ageing*. New York: Springer Publishing Company.

Touhy, T. & Jett, K. (2012). *Ebersole & Hess' Toward Healthy Ageing: Human Needs & Nursing Response*: St Louis: Elsevier Mosby.

Wadensten, B. (2007). The theory of gerotranscendence as applied to gerontological nursing – Part I. *International Journal of Older People Nursing*, 2(4), 289–94.

2

The demographics and epidemiology of ageing in the context of the changing needs of older adults

Marguerite Bramble

Learning objectives

After reading this chapter you will be able to:

1 Outline epidemiological frameworks in the context of older adults.

2 Describe major ageing demographic changes in the 20th and 21st centuries.

3 Describe the changing care needs of older adults as they age.

4 Discuss the unique needs of the old-old related to their quality of life, ability to function and perception of health and morale.

5 Discuss the principles of geriatric evaluation as a basis for strengths-based care and assessment in gerontological nursing.

Senescence
Physiological progressive deterioration of body systems that can increase mortality risk in an older person.

Epidemiology
The study of health amongst populations.

Ageing demographics
Statistical data relating to the ageing population and particular cohorts within it.

Introduction

Chapter 1 discussed ageing theories and gerontology and the importance for nurses in practice to understand the developmental processes of ageing when caring for older adults as they transition into old age and **senescence**. In this chapter we will discuss **epidemiology** and **ageing demographics** in the context of the changing and complex needs of older adults as they transition through the lifespan. Major policy changes in Australia and New Zealand relevant to nursing practice will also be included.

The epidemiology of ageing

The epidemiology of ageing helps nurses to understand changing patterns of health and disease in older populations. In order to identify causes and **risk factors** associated with disease, epidemiology uses two measures: firstly the measure of **morbidity**, which is defined as the **incidence** or risk associated with exposure to a disease, and secondly the measure of **prevalence**, or the number of people affected by a disease in a given population (Gordis, 2004). Ageing risk factors are associated with an increased risk of developing more complex disease patterns as one chronologically ages. These ageing risk factors are multidimensional and can be demographic, behavioural, biomedical, genetic, environmental, social or other **co-morbidity factors**, which can act independently or in combination. It is important for nurses in practice to understand the implications of the increasing incidence and prevalence of complex and **chronic disease** pathologies in older adults as they age. These complexities associated with ageing will be discussed in the frameworks of clinical epidemiology and life course epidemiology (Kuh et al., 2003).

Clinical epidemiology provides us with a framework and historical context for understanding the disease related 'epidemiological transition' from the 19th to 21st centuries across the human lifespan. In the 19th century there was a rapid decline in the **mortality** of infants and children from infectious diseases. In the 20th century there was an increase in life expectancy of adults and the young-old as a result of better management of conditions that affect multiple organ systems, described as cardiac, vascular, stroke, obesity, diabetes, hypertension and lung disease. In the 21st century, survival from management of systemic conditions has resulted in an increase in the prevalence of chronic degenerative diseases, particularly in the **old-old**, or those aged 85 years and over (Fillit, Rockwood & Woodhouse, 2010). Chronic degenerative conditions are mainly associated with the brain, such as dementia, Parkinson's disease, gait slowing and sensory loss.

The life course, or lifespan approach to epidemiology and disease prevention, supports the discussion in Chapter 1 that illness and disability may arise either as an accumulation of risk as one ages or as exposure to risk factors at

Risk factor(s)
Behaviour(s) that increase risk of disease.

Morbidity
Increasing risk of exposure to disease.

Incidence Risk associated with disease.

Prevalence
Percentage of the population affected by a disease or condition.

Co-morbidity factors
Factors that increase risk of developing chronic disease, such as depression.

Chronic disease
A disease that is persistent or otherwise long-lasting in its effects. The term 'chronic' is usually applied when the course of the disease lasts for more than three months.

Mortality The measure of the risk of disease severity.

Old-old People aged 85 years and above.

critical periods across a person's lifespan (Kuh et al., 2003). In an ageing population therefore, with a higher life expectancy and prevalence of associated risk factors, disability and chronic diseases will also become more prevalent (Australian Institute of Health and Welfare, 2006). Epidemiological data already have predicted that, as Australian populations age, and people survive longer with successfully managed chronic diseases of the circulatory and respiratory systems, dementia and related neurodegenerative disorders will become more prevalent and have a greater impact on their health and well-being (Access Economics, 2005; Australian Institute of Health and Welfare, 2004). In response to these changes governments have developed ageing policies that focus on health promotion to positively influence health behaviours at all ages. The intent of social and government policy is to provide health services that encourage healthy ageing and to prevent or delay the development of disability and chronic disease.

The demographics of ageing

Understanding current and future trends in ageing demographics provides a basis for nurses to plan care for individual groups and to recognise diverse cultural needs and responses to care provision. It is important to remember when reflecting on care needs that population ageing as a result of increasing life expectancy is a global phenomenon and is a positive indicator of improving global health for older people, both in developing and developed countries. In the first half of the 21st century it is predicted that the world's population aged 60 years and over will more than triple from 600 million to 2 billion (World Health Organization, 2013). The fastest growing group of the older population is that aged 80 and older and it is predicted that this group will quadruple to 400 million worldwide by 2050, with 100 million in China alone (World Health Organization, 2013).

Major ageing population trends: Australia and New Zealand

The statistics for population ageing in New Zealand and Australia show similar increasing trends in life expectancy, reflected by increasing percentages of those 85 years and over and 100 years and over in our populations (Hunter, 2012).

The most significant trend is the number of people living to 100 years of age. This group is projected to grow at the rate of more than 20 times that of the total population by 2050 (Touhy & Jett, 2012).

A snapshot of major demographic projections is presented to compare trends in older people (65 years and over) generally to those in the old-old age group, including the estimated number of centenarians.

1   In 2010 the percentage of the population aged 65 years and over in Australia was 13.3 per cent in 2010, while in New Zealand it was 12.1 per cent. In both countries the proportion of people 65 years and over is projected to increase to between 26 per cent and 28 per cent of the total population by 2051 (Australian Bureau of Statistics, 2008; Statistics New Zealand, 2007).

2   It is projected that by 2051 the 85 years and over aged group as a percentage of those aged 65 years and over will be 20 per cent in Australia and 24 per cent in New Zealand. By 2056 it is projected that there will be 71 200 centenarians in Australia and 153 800 in the 90 years and over aged group in New Zealand by 2051 (Australian Bureau of Statistics, 2008; Statistics New Zealand, 2007).

Ageing demographics in indigenous populations

The rapidly changing ageing demographic landscape in Australia and New Zealand also has implications for the issues concerning older people from indigenous populations. For indigenous Australians life expectancy at birth in 2001 was 17 years less than life expectancy for Australians as a whole. In indigenous populations the major factors influencing reduced life expectancy are the rising prevalence of chronic disease, disadvantaged socio-economic status and remoteness from health care services (Australian Institute of Health and Welfare, 2011). These risk factors have resulted in premature ageing, significantly different functional capabilities and eligibility for aged care services for indigenous Australians from the time they are 50 years and over (Australian Institute of Health and Welfare, 2007). Demographic data also show that indigenous older Australians have particular social and community needs in relation to staying in their communities, close to home and country, mainly in rural and remote areas.

In Australia these statistics highlight the need for nurses to consider development of best practice guidelines for indigenous populations, including Torres Strait Islanders. All clients of health services should be asked if they are of Aboriginal and/or Torres Strait Islander origin in the process of routine data collection. Despite improvements in recent years, there have been continuing problems in establishing and maintaining standard practice in the collection of indigenous status, resulting in the under-identification of Aboriginal and Torres Strait Islander people in key national health data sets (Australian Institute of Health and Welfare, 2010).

Similarly in New Zealand Maori life expectancy at birth from 2005 to 2007 was 7.9 years less for females and 8.6 years less for males than that for the non-Maori population (Ministry of Social Development New Zealand, 2010). As in Australia older Maoris are included in ageing demographic statistics from 50 years and over and are eligible for aged care services. Geographical accessibility in New Zealand has allowed for more successful services to be developed and provided for the Maori population. These services are supported by positive social and cultural attitudes to ageing in Maori communities which generally associate age with status and 'mana' (Ministry of Social Development New Zealand, 2010).

Ageing demographics in culturally and linguistically diverse populations

Older people from culturally and linguistically diverse (CALD) populations comprised one in three older Australians in 2006 (Australian Institute of Health and Welfare, 2007). CALD older people were most commonly born in Italy, Greece, Germany, the Netherlands and China. In the same year in New Zealand 27 per cent of older people were born overseas, most commonly from the UK, Asia, the Pacific Islands and North-west Europe (Statistics New Zealand, 2007). These statistics reflect the diversity of CALD populations in each country, and highlight the high degree of cultural competence and cultural

Culturally competent
Responding effectively to cultural and linguistic needs of clients and caregivers.

safety required from nurses in practice. To reduce health inequality in CALD populations both Australian and New Zealand national governments and nursing bodies have mandated the delivery of **culturally competent** nursing care (Nursing and Midwifery Board of Australia, 2011; Nursing Council of New Zealand, 2011). In practice nurses play a critical role in ensuring that the health sector forms partnerships with ethnic communities in developing culturally appropriate health promotion and health service delivery for older people (National Health and Medical Research Council, 2006).

The baby boomers cohort

From 2011 the baby boomers cohort, or those born between 1946 and 1964, have begun to turn 65. This large segment (approximately 24%) of the population brings with it unprecedented increases in population ageing. Nurses in practice will be integral to developing services that involve meeting the higher expectations of people in this segment, many of whom have reasonably high disposable income, are well educated and have often occupied positions of influence (Royal Australasian College of Physicians, 2011). In recognition of these changes the Australian government established the Ageing Well, Ageing Productively Program with the goal to achieve an additional 10 years of healthy life expectancy by 2050 for all Australians (Andrews & DOHA, 2001; Anstey et al., 2010; Anstey et al., 2011). In New Zealand the Health of Older People Strategy and the New Zealand Positive Ageing Strategy were developed to promote supporting older people to make age-related living choices and to enable a good quality of life in the community (Ramage, 2006).

These demographic statistics alone highlight the need for increasingly targeted services for the baby boomer cohort with the aim to extend healthy ageing and prevent the consequences of disabilities and chronic disease associated with ageing (Hunter, 2012).

Demographic statistics and epidemiological studies as the basis for practice

In response to population ageing, contemporary multidisciplinary research studies combine epidemiology data and demographic statistics to improve understanding of this complex area in practice. Findings from these studies also inform government policy and service delivery, and provide the basis for nurses to develop new practice models of care. When developing new models nurses in practice play a critical role in providing assessment data within these frameworks on risk factors and determinants for disability and chronic disease.

Using a demographic and epidemiological framework also assists nurses to identify non-modifiable and modifiable influences on a person's health and well-being as they age. Non-modifiable demographic factors are classified as age, gender, indigenous status, ethnic background, family history and genetic make-up. Modifiable epidemiological risk factors are classified as behavioural and biomedical. Major behavioural risk factors are described as tobacco smoking, excess alcohol use, physical inactivity, poor diet and other individual lifestyle factors, such as sexual behaviour and drug use. Biomedical risk factors are described as excess weight, high blood pressure, high blood cholesterol and other factors such as high blood glucose. Risk factors and determinants for disability and chronic disease are summarised in Table 2.1. A range of studies that increase our understanding of epidemiological and demographic ageing in the baby boomer and old-old cohorts are presented in the following sections.

TABLE 2.1 *Risk factors and determinants for disability and chronic disease*

BROAD INFLUENCES		MODIFIABLE RISK FACTORS	
Non-modifiable	**May or may not be modifiable**	**Behavioural**	**Biomedical**
Age	Socio-environmental factors	Tobacco smoking	Excess weight
Gender	Psychosocial factors	Excess alcohol use	High blood pressure
Indigenous status	Early life factors	Physical inactivity	High blood cholesterol
Ethnic background	Political factors	Poor diet	Other
Family history		Other	
Genetic make-up			

Source: with permission from the Australian Institute of Health and Welfare , *Chronic Diseases and Associated Risk Factors in Australia*, 2006, p. 13

Projections of causes of disability and ageing

The Dynamic Analyses to Optimise Ageing (DYNOPTA) study combines Australia wide demographic and longitudinal studies of ageing to generate epidemiological projections of expected health and morbidity within the baby boomer cohort (Anstey et al., 2011). These longitudinal data allow for analysis of prevalence, incidence and change in major causes of disability among people as they age (Anstey et al., 2011). The DYNOPTA study also provides new estimates of the prevalence of disease and disability based on larger numbers of the old-old than has previously been possible. As discussed in previous sections with the successful management of systemic diseases, the old-old are increasingly susceptible to conditions associated with the brain and mental health, such as dementia. This and other studies increase nurses' understanding of the unique needs and experiences of the old-old and how to achieve successful ageing using the strengths-based approach (see Chapter 3).

Mental health and cognitive decline in the old-old

As more people reach the 85 years and over and 100 years and over age groups, it is important for nurses in practice to build a knowledge base of their complex and multidimensional needs. Research studies achieve this by utilising the disability framework summarised in Table 2.1 combined with epidemiological indicators particularly important in these groups, such as functioning, memory and problem-solving ability. One such study found that decreased problem-solving ability and admission to residential care were related to greater depressive symptoms in these age groups (Margrett et al., 2010). Cognitive and problem-solving ability had the strongest influence on mental health, which led to a greater need for caregiving services. Another study found that psychological abilities play a more important influence on the need for social support than functional health and economic resources (MacDonald et al., 2010). These study findings demonstrate the need to examine a variety of factors which influence mental health and wellbeing in later life and to consider the unique contexts and differential experiences of the old-old (Margrett et al., 2010).

In the context of examining factors such as cognitive decline and depression in the old-old, it is important that nurses have the capability to assess a person's overall **quality of life** (QOL). Recent research has shown that, despite their incapacities, overall the old-old consider that they have a reasonably high QOL and individuals perceive their QOL better than nurses and caregivers do. This difference in subjects' and caregivers' perception is more pronounced for people with dementia and there is evidence that decreased QOL is more strongly influenced by depressive symptoms than by dementia severity (Lapid et al., 2011).

Quality of life
An individual's perception of their position in life in the context of the culture and value systems in which they live and in relation to their goals, expectations, standards and concerns.

These findings are supported by a third study which concluded that a large proportion of the old-old had high morale (von Heideken Wågert et al., 2005).

The most important factors for high morale were the absence of depressive symptoms, living in ordinary housing, not feeling lonely and a low number of chronic ailments. The study found that those living in residential and nursing homes had a shorter survival when aged 90 years and above. This suggests that even at the very oldest ages, the majority preferred to live at home (von Heideken Wågert et al., 2005).

Other major impacts for nurses to consider of age-related changes in cognitive and functional status in the old-old are:

Geriatric syndrome
Occurs when the unique features of common health conditions in the elderly, such as delirium, falls, incontinence and frailty, are highly prevalent, multifactorial, and associated with substantial morbidity and poor outcomes.

- Those who are termed old-old are increasingly susceptible to **geriatric syndrome**, or a complex combination of age related changes such as multiple co-morbidities, cognitive impairment, frailty and disability. This results in an increasing risk of falls, delirium and incontinence (Royal Australasian College of Physicians, 2011).

- Falls have been identified as a national health priority in Australia and account for 90 per cent of fractures in the old-old. Falls and the resulting injuries are major reasons for admission to residential aged care facilities. The social costs from fear of falling may be debilitating and lead to severe restrictions on a person's level of functioning and social interaction, chronic pain, increasing loss of independence and reduction in well-being (Bradley, 2013).

- The risk of delirium increases with advancing age, and is more likely to occur in the old-old, in those with dementia and those who have been prescribed psychoactive medications. The Australian government has committed to improving health care of people with dementia by adopting dementia as the ninth National Health Priority Area in 2012.

- This age group is also vulnerable to hospital admission due to episodes of acute illness and disability and their informal carers are vulnerable to social losses, stress, depression, poor health and economic loss.

In summary, due to the increasing **complexity** and changing needs of the old-old, many lose their ability to live independently because of limited mobility, frailty or other physical or mental health problems. Many require long-term

Complexity
Focus on multiple spheres of physical, functional, psychological and social care.

care, including home-based nursing, community, institutional (residential) and hospital-based care. Although family continues to provide the majority of care to their older relatives most experience a period of dependence and a need for care beyond what families can provide before the end of life (Koch & Garratt, 2001).

Contemporary models of nursing care need to take into account major physical, psychological and social transitions that occur, particularly for the old-old, and foster the health and participation of older people in their care. Evidence-based nursing models currently under development for older people and their families are based on strengths-based assessment, case management and transitional approaches from community to long-term care. These models will be further discussed in Chapter 3.

The multidimensional needs-based approach

Nurses in practice must have a sound understanding of the multidimensional and changing needs of older people in the context of ageing based on demographic and epidemiological frameworks. Epidemiological data show that as people age there is an increased incidence, or risk, of co-morbidities, such as mental disorders, bone and joint disorders, visual impairment, blindness, hearing impairment, oral disease and neurological and genetic disorders (Chang & Johnson, 2008). Acute disease conditions can also present concurrently with chronic illness, resulting in increasing complexity (Australian Institute of Health & Welfare, 2006).

However it is also important to remember, as discussed in previous sections, that in the context of overall health older people are fitter than they were in previous decades and it is a widely perpetuated myth that it is too late for them to benefit from changing lifelong unhealthy habits (Burbank, Padula & Nigg, 2000; Fillit et al., 2010). Many health problems exhibited in older people are the result of modifiable lifestyle choices identified in Table 2.1 and resultant chronic diseases tend to develop over many years. Nurses have the opportunity therefore to promote the development of healthy habits and intervene to prevent chronic disease and neurodegenerative conditions by working with older people and their strengths. This strengths-based approach to care will be introduced in Chapter 3 and further explored in later chapters.

When assessing older people nurses must take into account multidimensional physical, mental, emotional and spiritual needs in order to improve quality of life. Their goal is to maximise the older adult's independence and function by recognising strengths in the context of normal ageing changes, the client's past health history and history of present illness. They should also actively involve older adults and family members as much as possible in the decision making process about care. Reluctance to accord older people appropriate recognition for their strengths and capabilities indicates a failure to understand the needs of the older adult (Butler, Lewis & Sunderland, 1998). These principles of assessment form the basis of strengths-based care that are presented in Chapter 3.

As discussed in Chapter 1 the scope of the gerontological nurse is to ensure that a comprehensive geriatric needs evaluation is provided to fully assess the complex needs of older clients within three underlying principles:

1 Physical, psychological and socio-economic factors interact in complex ways to influence the health and functional status of the older person.
2 Comprehensive evaluation of an older person's health status requires an assessment in each of these domains.
3 Functional abilities should be a central focus of the comprehensive evaluation. Other more traditional measures of health, such as medical diagnosis, nursing assessment and physical examination results, form the basic foundation for the assessment in order to determine overall health, well-being and the need for social services (Kane, Ouslander & Abrass, 2004).

There are other influences in addition to normal ageing changes, chronic disease processes and environmental influences that may impact on comprehensive nursing assessment for older people. These are: communication difficulties caused by decreased vision or hearing; slow speech or English as a second language resulting in under-reporting of symptoms; and vague or non-specific complaints associated with cognitive impairment and co-morbidities such as depression and social isolation (Tabloski, 2010). In a holistic care framework nurses are in a position to identify current or potential health problems within the context of normal ageing changes and each individual's life and health goals.

In the context of the multidimensional needs of older people nursing assessment should also take into account functional health patterns such as health management, nutrition, elimination, activity and sleep, cognition and self-perception, role, sexuality, values and beliefs, and coping and stress (Tabloski, 2010). Additional areas to be considered are: health promotion and disease prevention, for example pathology and cancer screening and vaccinations; finances; driving status and safety record; and social supports (family, caregiver stress, safety of living environment). This usually involves coordinating input and advice from various health professionals in the multidisciplinary team to achieve a coordinated and integrated care plan. This multidisciplinary approach, particularly if adopted in primary care settings, is associated with a reduction in hospital admissions for older people (Tabloski, 2010).

ultidimensional functional assessment

Case scenario 2.1

Alice Jones is 86 and lives at home with her 87 year old husband Clem, who is experiencing general good health for his age. Two months ago Alice fell in the bathroom and sustained a deep skin tear to her right ankle. Clem, who was unable to lift Alice, rang the ambulance and she was taken to hospital. She spent a week in the acute medical ward for assessment and review. The initial assessment identified that three months ago Alice started experiencing dizzy spells. Until this time she had enjoyed reasonably good health, as her hypertension and type 2 diabetes were well managed by her general practitioner. The assessment also identified her blood pressure and blood sugar levels as unstable, she was still experiencing dizziness when mobilising and there were some signs of cognitive decline and overall sadness, as described by Alice. She was transferred to the subacute extended care unit for ongoing assessment of her overall functional status and management of her ankle wound.

When Alice is admitted to the extended care unit you, as a registered nurse, have been asked to update Alice's functional assessment as part of her geriatric evaluation. When approaching Alice, who is sitting in a chair next to her bed, you note that she looks tired and withdrawn but she immediately smiles when you approach her.

Subacute extended care unit Distinct unit located within an acute care general hospital that utilises licensed long-term care beds.

Reflective questions
Read and reflect on the case scenario of Alice and address the following questions:

› Based on the epidemiological data provided in this chapter what are the major factors to consider when updating Alice's functional assessment?

› What influences would Alice's age, underlying health problems and social and biographical history have on the factors to consider in your assessment?

› How would you assess or measure Alice's quality of life?

Reflective activity
You are a registered nurse providing caring for Alice in the subacute extended care unit.

● Has your nursing education included identifying your scope of practice in providing care for old-old clients such as Alice?
● Can you think of situations where staff mentors have outlined these requirements when you have commenced on a new ward setting?

Summary

Demographic and epidemiological studies inform nursing knowledge about the complex and changing needs of older people as they age.

- Studies of the old-old provide valuable insights into their unique needs related to quality of life, ability to function, overall perception of health and morale.
- These findings assist in developing health services and models of practice for the unprecedented number of old-old baby boomers in the future.
- Nurses' scope of practice is to provide comprehensive geriatric evaluation and holistic care based on an individual client's needs.

Conclusion

This chapter has outlined major ageing changes in the 21st century. Caring for our ageing population is now a government priority in both Australia and New Zealand as costs of health care for older people escalate. Government driven multidisciplinary ageing research studies are imperative to increase our understanding of the changing patterns of health and the risks associated with ageing, disability and illness in our older population. New knowledge of emerging patterns in the old-old assists nurses in practice to fully assess their strengths and complex needs. Nurses can also work with older clients to change unhealthy life habits and assist in preventing, or reducing the risk of, multiple co-morbidities of ageing. Nursing multidimensional assessment and evaluation provides the framework for strengths-based models of care.

Further reading

You may like to take a look at the following reading recommendations:

- Australia – Department of Health: http://www.health.gov.au/
- Australian Institute of Health and Welfare: http://www.aihw.gov.au/
- New Zealand Ageing Statistics: http://www.stats.govt.nz
- New Zealand – Ministry of Social Development. The report 'An Ageing Population' is available at: https://www.msd.govt.nz/what-we-can-do/seniorcitizens/positive-ageing/trends/ageing-population.html

References

Access Economics. (2005). *Dementia Estimates and Projections: Australian States and Territories. Report for Alzheimer's Australia*. Canberra.

Andrews, K. & DOHA. (2001). *National Strategy for and Ageing Australia: An Older Australia, Challenges and Opportunities for All*. Canberra: DOHA.

Anstey, K., Birrell, C., Browning, C., Burns, R., Byles, J., Kiely, K., ... Ross, L. (2011). Understanding ageing in older Australians: The contribution of the Dynamic Analyses to Optimise Ageing (DYNOPTA) project to the evidence base and policy. *Australasian Journal on Ageing*, 30 (October), 24–31.

Anstey, K., Byles, J., Luszcz, M., Mitchell, P., Steel, D., Booth, H., ... Kendig, H. (2010). Cohort profile: The Dynamic Analyses to Optimize Ageing (DYNOPTA) project. *International Journal of Epidemiology*, 39(1), 44–51.

Australian Bureau of Statistics. (2008). *Population Projections, Australia, 2006 to 2101*. Canberra.

Australian Institute of Health and Welfare. (2004). *The Impact of Dementia on the Health and Aged Care Systems*. Canberra.

Australian Institute of Health and Welfare. (2006). *Chronic Diseases and Associated Risk Factors in Australia*. Canberra.

Australian Institute of Health and Welfare. (2007). *Older Australians at a Glance*. (4th edition). Canberra.

Australian Institute of Health and Welfare. (2010). *National Best Practice Guidelines for Collecting Indigenous Status in Health Data Sets*. Canberra.

Australian Institute of Health and Welfare. (2011). *Life Expectancy and Mortality of Aboriginal and Torres Strait Islander People*. Canberra.

Bradley, C. (2013). *Trends in Hospitalisations Due to Falls by Older People, Australia 1999–00 to 2010–11*. Canberra: AIHW.

Burbank, P., Padula, C. & Nigg, C. (2000). Changing health behaviour of older adults. *Gerontological Nursing*, 26(3), 26–33.

Butler, R., Lewis, M. & Sunderland, T. (1998). *Aging and Mental Health*. Austin: PRO-ED.

Chang, E. & Johnson, A. (2008). *Chronic Illness and Disability: Principles for Nursing Practice*. Chatswood: Elsevier.

Fillit, H., Rockwood, K. & Woodhouse, K. (2010). *Textbook of Geriatric Medicine and Gerontology*. Philadelphia: Elsevier.

Gordis, L. (2004). *Epidemiology*. (3rd edition). Philadelphia: Elsevier Saunders.

Hunter, S. (2012). *Miller's Nursing for Wellness in Older Adults*. Philadelphia: Wolters Kluwer/Lippincott Williams & Wilkins.

Kane, R., Ouslander, J. & Abrass, I. (2004). *Essentials of Clinical Geriatrics*. (5th edition). New York: McGraw-Hill.

Koch, S. & Garratt, S. (2001). *Assessing Older People*. Sydney: Maclennan & Petty.

Kuh, D., Ben-Shlomo, Y., Lynch, J., Hallqvist, J. & Power, C. (2003). Life course epidemiology. *Journal of Epidemiology and Community Health*, 57(10), 778–83.

Lapid, M., Rummans, T., Boeve, J., McCormick, J., Pankratz, V. , Cha, R., ... Petersen, R. (2011). What is the quality of life in the oldest old? *International Psychogeriatrics*, 23(6), 1003–10.

MacDonald, M., Aneja, A., Martin, P., Margrett, J. & Poon, L. (2010). Distal and proximal resource influences on economic dependency among the oldest old. *Gerontology*, 56, 100–5.

Margrett, J., Martin, P., Woodard, J., Miller, L., Macdonald, M., Baenziger, J., ... the Georgia Centenarian Study (2010). Depression among centenarians and the oldest old: Contributions of cognition and personality. *Gerontology*, 56(1), 93–9.

Ministry of Social Development New Zealand. (2010). *The Social Report 2010*. Wellington.

National Health and Medical Research Council. (2006). *Cultural Competency in Health: A Guide for Policy, Partnerships and Participation*. Canberra: Australian Government.

Nursing Council of New Zealand. (2011). *Guidelines for Cultural Safety, the Treaty of Waitangi and Maori Health in Nursing Education and Practice*. Wellington.

Nursing and Midwifery Board of Australia. (2011). *Code of Ethics for Nurses*. Melbourne.

Ramage, C. (2006). *Evaluation of Strategies for Ageing in Place*. Auckland: The University of Auckland.

Royal Australasian College of Physicians. (2011). *Geriatric Medicine Advanced Training Curriculum*. Sydney.

Statistics New Zealand. (2007). *New Zealand's 65+ Population: A Statistical Volume*. Wellington.

Tabloski, P. (2010). *Gerontological Nursing*. (2nd edition). New Jersey: Pearson.

Touhy, T. & Jett, K. (2012). *Ebersole & Hess' Toward Healthy Ageing: Human Needs & Nursing Response*: St Louis: Elsevier.

von Heideken Wågert, P., Rönnmark, B., Rosendahl, E., Lundin-Olsson, L. & Gustavsson, J. (2005). Morale in the oldest old: The Umeå 85+ study. *Age and Ageing*, 34(3), 249–55.

World Health Organization. (2013). *World Health Statistics 2013*. Geneva.

Principles of strengths-based care and other nursing models

3

Wendy Moyle

Learning objectives

After reading this chapter you will be able to:

1 Identify the advantages of nursing models to guide nursing practice.

2 Define the key components of strengths-based nursing care.

3 Discuss how to use the strengths-based approach in nursing practice.

4 Define the key components of person-centred, relationship-centred care and the Capabilities Model of Dementia Care.

5 Examine the relationship between the models outlined and their relationship to practice.

Introduction

Although there is great interest in how to provide the best quality of care to older people, there are few well-defined **nursing models** of care to guide practice. A nursing model of care provides the framework on which nursing care can focus and influences the way that care is provided. Pearson, Vaughan and Fitzgerald (2005, p. 29) outline the basic components or building blocks of a nursing model as:

> **Nursing models** The frameworks on which nursing care can focus.

1 The beliefs and values on which the model is based.
2 The theories and concepts on which it is built.

Furthermore, Pearson and colleagues (2005) argue that nursing models are necessary to:

1 Guide nursing practice as models lead to consistency in care.
2 Reduce conflict within the care team.
3 Make sense of the nursing care given and therefore allow the care to be understood by all health care professionals, as well as patients and their families.

4　Give direction to nursing care.

5　Act as a guide to decision and policy making.

6　Give purpose and guidance to choosing team members.

Support for nursing models of care predominately comes from the US where the development of nursing models and their use in care has been well defined for many years in the literature. Popular models of care include **King's Model** of Care, which focuses on the importance of interaction (King, 1997) and **Orem's Model**, which focuses on the concept of self-care and integrates the theory of human needs (Orem, 1987).

King's Model
A nursing model of care that focuses on the importance of interaction.

Orem's Model
A nursing model of care that focuses on the concept of self-care and integrates the theory of human needs.

Team nursing Involves the use of a team leader and team members who deliver care to a group of patients.

Primary nursing care
Comprehensive, individualised care performed by the same nurse.

In Australia and New Zealand nursing practice has tended to concentrate on nursing models of care delivery rather than theoretical models. For example, over the years the focus has been on **team nursing** and **primary nursing care** (Pearson et al., 2005). Team nursing originated in the 1950s and comprises a team leader and team members who provide various aspects of nursing care to a group of patients. This model of care delivery allows team members to deliver care they are component in and results in team members having distinct roles that they perform. The team leader must have good leadership skills to ensure the nursing group is truly working towards the same patient care goals. Team nursing is one of the most popular models, as it is effective in situations where the skill mix or experience is diverse. It allows junior nurses to undertake roles to fit their capabilities and senior nurses to mentor the juniors in their role, while completing skills appropriate to their competency base.

Primary nursing evolved in the 1970s and refers to comprehensive, individualised care performed by the same nurse. The primary nurse in this situation completes all care for a small group of patients and communicates the patient's status to the health care team. A higher number of registered nurses are needed in this model. Although both team nursing and primary nursing are popular models of nursing practice the current research is not conclusive in terms of the benefit of team or primary nursing to care outcomes. Little benefit has been found for the model of primary nursing and it is considered to be too costly to implement.

The majority of the models of care defined in the literature focus on the acute care situation, whereas to date there has been limited focus on models that can be used within subacute nursing/rehabilitation, community and long-term care. This chapter aims to highlight models that are appropriate for care of older people. The chapter describes **strengths-based care** and takes into account other models of care continuity such as person-centred, relationship-centred and the **Capabilities Model of Dementia Care** (CMDC). The chapter commences with a brief overview of **person-centred care**.

> **Strengths-based care** An approach to care that focuses on individuals' strengths rather than pathologies.
>
> **Capabilities Model of Dementia Care** A model of dementia care informed by the capabilities approach.
>
> **Person-centred care** Treatment and care provided by health services that places the person at the centre of their own care and considers the needs of the older person's carers.

Person-centred care

The last two decades have seen a growing emphasis on the uniqueness of the person and therefore the importance of customising care to the needs and wishes of the person. Dr Tom Kitwood at the University of Bradford, UK developed the concept of person-centred care in the late 1980s in relation to care of the older person with dementia. Although promoted for care of people with dementia the concepts are appropriate for all people receiving care. The primary principle of person-centred care is to redirect attention from the biomedical aspects of the disease to the subjective experience of the person with dementia. This approach supports the rights, values and beliefs of the person. The aim is to maximise the person's potential and to involve them in their care as well as in decision making about their care. This model supports the belief that there is meaning in the behaviours that the person exhibits and person-centred care has been shown to have a positive impact on the job satisfaction of staff (van den Pol-Grevelink et al., 2012).

The VIPS – main concepts of person-centred care

It is common for care staff not to be able to describe the concepts of person-centred care beyond that it is individualised care. Brooker (2007) developed the acronym **VIPS** to help explain the four main concepts of person-centred care and as a means of educating staff. These are:

> **VIPS** The four main concepts of person-centred care.

- V – a value base that asserts the value of all humans regardless of their age or cognitive ability.
- I – an individualised approach, which recognises the person as a unique human.

P – understanding of the world from the perspective of the person being cared for.

S – encouraging a social environment that supports the person's individu- alised needs.

Personhood is the central concept in person-centred care. Kitwood defined this as 'a standing or a status that is bestowed on one human being, by an-

Personhood The standing or status bestowed on a human being.

other in the context of relationship and social being' (Kitwood, 1997, p. 8). Furthermore, Kitwood (1997, p. 8) argued that per- sonhood accords people with dementia with an ethical status that offers them absolute value and as a consequence an obligation 'to treat each other with deep respect'. He stated that dementia is not necessarily a downward trajectory and argued that through good communication or, as he termed it 'positive people work', a person's condition may improve. Calling a person by their name, affirming their views and encouraging people to play in activities they enjoy is a form of positive people work that will engender a person-centred approach to care. The move to long-term care can undermine a person's sense of identity. Care that is truly person-centred, that understands the person's needs, including their values, is important.

Using a person-centred approach

Case scenario 3.1

Janet, an 85 year old former ballet teacher, lives in a long-term care facility because of increasing cognitive impairment due to a diagnosis of Alzheimer's disease. Janet complains to her family and staff that she is lonely and that she hates the long days spent sitting in front of the television. Although the facility offers a number of activities throughout the week, Janet has not shown an interest in any of them.

The staff decide to update Janet's social biography and when speaking with Janet and her family they find that she learnt ballet early in life and went on to dance in numerous performances. In her early 30s she accepted an appointment as a ballet teacher at a major ballet school where she taught for 25 years. Discussions with Janet reveal that her keen interest

in ballet continues and staff look for opportunities to re-engage her.

The first question she is asked is whether she'd like to attend a ballet performance. Janet tells the staff that she doesn't feel ready to go out in the evening to a performance. They encourage family and other staff members to bring in DVDs of ballets for Janet to watch. Staff and family also engage Janet in helping to develop a display of photographs of famous ballerinas and they ask the local ballet school to present an afternoon concert to residents, staff and family. Janet immediately shows interest in this activity and, rather than sitting in front of the television, takes an interest not only in these specific activities but also begins to attend music groups. The focus on ballet demonstrates a valuing of Janet, an individualised approach to activities that were based on her interest and helped to meet her social needs.

Reflective questions

Read and reflect on this case scenario and address the following questions:

> What was the trigger for staff to learn more about Janet?

> What changes in nursing practice have helped to change Janet's perception of involvement in activities?

> How does the involvement of ballet activities demonstrate a valuing of Janet?

> What are the advantages of using a person-centred approach to nursing care?

Butterworth (2012, p. 22) states that every member of the care team must have the same set of values to achieve person-centred care. A summary of these values is outlined below.

- Emphasising strengths and abilities rather than weaknesses and disabilities.
- Focusing on the perspective of the individual, rather than the staff's perspective.
- Promoting feelings of well-being and minimising feelings of ill-being.
- Seeing 'challenging' or 'problem' behaviour as an attempt at communication; the behaviour being a challenge or problem for others.
- Accepting that feelings are displayed as behaviours – with the onus on staff to interpret.
- Accepting the reality of the person and not insisting on bringing a person into the staff's reality, which can cause distress.
- Acknowledging that each person is a unique individual in all words and actions.
- Not using inappropriate behaviours and words, for example, those that infantilise, belittle, outpace, mock or ignore.
- Not using labels, for example, 'a wanderer', 'a spitter' or 'a feeder'.
- Not viewing a person as 'uncooperative' – this only means that the person does not want to do what staff want, when they want.
- Promoting dignity at all times, including using the person's name, rather than terms that may be patronising, for example, 'sweetie' and 'honeybun'. Acknowledging that person-centred care is the opposite of a task-orientated approach.
- Working with a person rather than 'doing to' a person.

Relationship-centred care

Relationship-centred care centres on the many important relationships present in the long-term care setting and the imperative to optimal care that relationships bring. Nolan and colleagues (2004) argue that there are three agencies involved in the care of the person with dementia –

> **Relationship-centred care**
> Centres on the importance of relationships.

the client, the family and the staff – and that each member is a valuable contributor to the care provision. Furthermore, quality care is argued to be dependent on the relationship between these groups. This approach recognises and values the mutual recognition between people and the opportunities offered through the secure foundations of knowing each other. Such relationships are essential when an individual has dementia as the knowledge created within the relationship allows gaps in the memory of the person with dementia to be partly filled. Furthermore, a relationship-centred approach is person oriented rather than task oriented. Caregiving is therefore centred on the needs of the person in the moment and how these needs can be met in the moment. For many people with dementia it is through these supportive relationships that they are able to enjoy quality of life.

The relationship-centred approach accentuates the role of interdependence and the importance this has in shaping our lives. This approach situates the person with dementia, their family and staff in a relational context, rather than one based on individuality, independence and autonomy. Here caregiving is understood within the context of relationship (Nolan et al., 2004) and interactions among people as the foundation of any therapeutic or healing activity (Tresolini & Pew-Fetzer Task Force, 1994, p. 11). Although the relationship-centred approach privileges personhood as essential to a model of quality dementia care, it equally values and embraces the need for mutual recognition and meaningful involvement that is derived through reciprocal care relationships (Nolan et al., 2004).

Relationship-centred care promotes an integrated approach to health care by uniting the psychological, social and biomedical aspects of health and by addressing the interdependencies between them (Aveyard & Davies, 2006). In this way a relationship-centred approach to dementia care acknowledges the biomedical aspects of dementia and the value this understanding can bring to the person with dementia while not privileging it above the equally (if not more) important psychosocial aspects of health.

The desire to provide a framework for nurses to practise and that would meet the needs of older people, their families and staff encouraged the development of the **Senses Framework**. Nolan and colleagues (2006) argued that nursing homes need to create an environment in which older people and staff experience six senses (see below). They viewed staff well-being as being essential for residents' quality of life and staff job satisfaction. The Senses Framework was developed over a 20 year period and concerns the relationships between family and formal carers.

> **Senses Framework**
> A framework that focuses on six senses.

The six senses are:

1 A sense of security: Feeling safe.
2 A sense of significance: Feeling you matter.
3 A sense of belonging: Having a 'place'.
4 A sense of purpose: Having a direction.
5 A sense of continuity: Linking the past, present and future.
6 A sense of fulfilment/achievement: To feel you're getting somewhere.

Capabilities Model of Dementia Care

The CMDC was conceptualised by Wendy Moyle (Cooke et al., 2013). The model is informed by the capabilities approach (Nussbaum, 2000, 2004) and research undertaken by Moyle and colleagues over a number of years, including testing of the model using a clinical trial approach (e.g. Cooke et al., 2013; Moyle et al., 2013a; Moyle et al., 2013b). The CMDC is underpinned by a conceptual framework that guides its practice in residential aged care facilities (RACFs). The framework comprises person-centred, relationship-centred and strengths-based approaches to care, each contributing to the way care is enacted. The essential aim of this model is to expand opportunities for people with dementia to achieve their conception of a 'life well lived'. The CMDC includes a list of 10 capabilities. These are considered fundamental opportunities to be made available to people with dementia in RACFs so that this aim is achievable.

The 10 capabilities in the new model of care basically reflect that a person with dementia should be able to:

1 Feel valued.
2 Experience the best health possible.

3 Live independently with compassionate support from important others.
4 Enjoy pleasurable experiences through senses, imagination and thought.
5 Experience and express emotion in a way that is true to oneself.
6 Reflect and decide on things that matter to oneself including plans for the future and end of life.
7 Experience connection with others where they can contribute and be contributed to and where there is self-respect, dignity and a sense of shared humanity with individuals and the wider community.
8 Live in a way where engaging with nature (plants, animals, sun, moon) is a natural part of life.
9 Play in a way that is meaningful and fun.
10 Experience a sense of control in how to live their life.

The capability 'feeling valued' is central to providing opportunities for people with dementia to 'live life well'. It is reflected in the person's ability to:

- Live one's own idea of a good life.
- Feel they are living and not simply waiting to die.
- Feel valued by others and not devalued because of their dementia.
- Live a life where their past, present and future are valued and accepted.

The capabilities approach belongs to theories of human flourishing (Jennings, 2000). Theories of human flourishing provide a valuable foundation to our understanding of quality of life (QOL) for people living with dementia. Importantly, they conceptualise QOL as a ceiling towards which caregiving efforts should be designed to strive rather than a minimum below which no significant societal expenditure is required (Jennings, 2000). Theories of human flourishing ratify the beliefs that disability, for example, as a result of a condition such as dementia is socially brokered, and advocates respect for people in such circumstances (Hooper, 2007). This approach arose as an alternative to utilitarian approaches to people welfare through the work of Amartya Sen, an economist and Martha Nussbaum, a lawyer and philosopher (Nussbaum & Sen, 1993).

The capability approach argues that disability (this can be related to anything from disease to poverty) can interfere with a person's ability to make choices, to be valued and to participate as a full member of society. Furthermore, this approach considers and sets the elements necessary to experience optimal well-being, as well as the standard by which we measure QOL. Nussbaum's work on capabilities argues that there are 10 capabilities that a 'good society' should ensure are available to all people. These capabilities are considered to be essential to 'living life well' (Nussbaum, 2004). Each capability resonates with what a person should be able to do and be and therefore under-pins the prerequisites of a just society and advocates a valuing of the individual choice. However, in this approach the choice that the individual makes is less important than the range of options that are encouraged by society. Therefore, in a capabilities approach the possibilities are other than the conventional op-portunities offered. The CMDC is guided by Nussbaum's ideas but reflects the dementia-specific nature of this model.

The 10 capabilities listed in the CMDC are considered fundamental op-portunities to be made 'available' to people with dementia. The list however is not prescriptive. Residents are able to choose whether to use these capabilities in their life; what is important is that their choice is a free choice, as opposed to one that is constrained by the available resources to the resident, most par-ticularly their ability to communicate and be heard by an advocate within their residence. It is therefore incumbent upon the aged care organisation (and soci-ety) to provide a care environment with the material and intellectual resources and commitment to actively support the person with dementia to achieve these capabilities.

Strengths-based nursing care

The strengths perspective comes from the discipline of social work (Staudt, Howard & Drake, 2001). Strengths-based care is an approach to care that helps move attention away from tasks and problems to simply seeing the person and their abilities. This is a different approach to nursing practice where the pre-vailing perspective is on helping. The belief has been that people need help because they have a problem, which sets them apart from other people who do not have the problem. An approach focused on problems relies on the need to find an expert to fix the problem while the person with the problem is not considered to be able to participate, control their problem or learn from their problem. This labelling of the person and the problem can in effect limit the options available. On the other hand the premise of strengths-based care is that every individual, family, group and community has strengths, and the focus needs to be on these strengths rather than pathology. The strengths-based ap-proach assumes patients will do better when they are helped to identify and to use their strengths and resources available to them. There is an assump-tion also that the community is a rich source of resources and that humans are capable of change and that learning occurs through reflection on change. Furthermore, the components nurses using a strengths-based delivery are most interested in are the essential collaboration between patient and nurse and the opportunity to empower people to take a lead in their own care process. The strengths approach focuses on the identification and use of an individual's strengths and resources to problem solve and effect change (Cox, 2001). To assist this change the nurse must acknowledge and value the patient's beliefs, their prior experiences and concerns to assist a positive health journey.

Strengths theory highlights the individual's characteristics, capabilities and behaviours as being unique and therefore nurses must listen, observe and understand the person in order to appreciate their strengths. Too often in practice older people are discarded as being old and therefore unable to do things for themselves. The care in this context becomes 'doing for' rather than 'doing with' the older person and is not satisfying for the older person or care staff. When working within the strengths-based perspective the nurse uses their strengths to discover, affirm and enhance the capabilities, interests, knowledge, goals and resources of older persons (Saleebey, 1996, 2000, 2002).

Strengths perspective in care of older people

When using a strengths-based model of care caregivers work with the older person, their family and other staff to determine their strengths and abilities. They also focus on how the environment can help maintain or improve these (Feeley & Gottlieb, 2000). This approach recognises that, in spite of an apparent poor functioning ability of older people, they retain valuable lifelong abilities that enable them to do things independently, or with varying degrees of help (Fast & Chapin, 2000). This philosophy encourages the opinion that older people retain more than they have lost and therefore people should be encouraged to do things independently for as long as possible to optimise independence. Such an approach in practice aims to encourage life satisfaction and to reduce caregiver burden. Furthermore, this approach is one of collaboration and partnership between the nurse and patient. The tenets of a strengths-based approach and techniques to implement such an approach are outlined in Table 3.1.

A strengths-based approach is useful when implementing health promotion as it encourages interest in the patient's own health, the actions people take to help each other to cope, and healthy environments or creating healthy

TABLE 3.1 *Techniques to assist a strengths-based approach into practice*

TENET	TECHNIQUES
Self-determination	Provide opportunities for patients to discuss their strengths, capabilities and areas that they would like to expand upon. Focus on what the patients want to improve their well-being.
Empowerment	Provide patients with opportunities to use their skills, strengths and capabilities so that they feel they have control over their situation.
Collaboration	Provide opportunities for patients to work together with their family, staff or other patients/residents on a mutually agreed activity. This will encourage the individual and/or group to use their skills to the best advantage.
Reflection on change	Provide opportunities for staff to become familiar with patients' stories and use these to mutually identify areas for future development. Such opportunities can occur in one-on-one sessions, group sessions and reading written biographies.
Community engagement	Encourage patients, staff and families to participate in community networking through local events. Where patients have strengths in community engagement, encourage active participation.
Regeneration	Encourage sharing of success. Encourage patients, families and staff to share stories that may also help others develop successful goals.

Source: Adapted from Fast & Chapin, 2000; and Saleebey, 2002

environments that assist with good health. The strengths-based approach also aims to collaborate with patients and their families' functioning and strengths in the belief that they have unique talents and skills as well as unmet needs (Rashid & Ostermann, 2009). Nurses working within a strengths-based approach emphasise strengths-based assessment to assess the skills, competencies and characteristics of patients and their families. Strengths-based assessment uses tools that assess emotional and behavioural skills, competencies and characteristics. One such way to identify strengths rather than focus on the identification of problems and pathology is to use the ROPES Model (Graybeal, 2001). This acronym stands for 'Resources, Opportunities, Possibilities, Exceptions and Solutions' (Table 3.2). The nurse can interview the patient and family member to gather appropriate assessment information.

The growing number of older people requires us to think differently about their potential care and support requirements. Strengths-based care offers the opportunity for older people, their families, carers and communities to support and encourage them in identifying and mobilising their strengths and resources. By doing so they can live a life that encourages empowerment and quality of life. Such an approach requires attention from agencies and care providers to system change processes as well as a change in attitudes and values that offers co-partnership between health care providers and clients.

TABLE 3.2 *How the ROPES Model can be used for assessment*

THE ROPES ASSESSMENT	
Resources	What personal, family, social, organisational and community resources does the patient have?
Options	What options are available in terms of focus and choice?
	What can be accessed? What is available?
Possibilities	What possibilities are available in terms of the patient's future?
	Focus, their imagination, creativity, vision of the future, a play? What has been thought of but not tried?
Exceptions	When is the problem not happening? When is the problem different? How has person survived, endured, thrived?
Solutions	The nurse must focus on constructing solutions not solving problems. Ask: What's working now? What are the successes? What would the patient like to continue? What would the patient want to do if a miracle occurred? What can the patient do to create a miracle?

Source: Graybeal, 2001, p. 237

Using a strengths-based approach to make change

Case scenario 3.2

Ron, an 80 year old man, who was living in a long-term care environment because of his increasing frailty, spent his days either sitting in a chair watching television or asleep on his bed. He often complained to staff and family that he was of no use any more and that he was waiting for Heaven's doors to open for him. While staff were kind to Ron and recognised that he was bored, they accepted that he was old and he had little to offer.

June, a new graduate, was hard working and wanted to make a difference. She spent time with Ron acknowledging that she was ready to listen, and soon learnt he was a former chairperson of a large board, with a background in accounting. He felt valued while in this role and his move into a nursing home had removed this role and his feeling of being valued. June acknowledged that, although he was physically frail, his mind was active and his strengths in leadership and accounting could assist other residents.

With Ron's agreement June helped set up a weekly residents' meeting with Ron in the chairperson's role. One of the residents, a former secretary, agreed to take minutes of the meeting. In a very short time the residents were directing the changes they wanted via the meeting and the group cohesion spurred them on. Ron was no longer watching television or sleeping during the day; he was preparing for the next meeting. He reported back to Joan that his life again had meaning.

Reflective questions

Read and reflect on the case example of Ron and address the following questions:

> Have you come across patients/residents who also don't feel valued?

> Do you know what helps them to feel valued?

> When next in this situation consider how you might encourage a strengths-based model of care.

Reflective activity

Consider your nursing education and practice and think about the following:

- How were nursing models presented to you in your nursing education? Did this knowledge influence your practice?
- Do you see examples of nursing models of care in practice? If so what are the models you have seen? Did clinical staff or your instructor outline the model of care when you started working in a new ward?
- How does the strengths-based approach fit with current clinical practice? Can you think of situations where this approach might have been used to guide your nursing practice?

Summary

- Nursing models of care differ from one another although they all demonstrate the values and beliefs on which practice is based.
- They encourage a continuity of care that is understood by all who practise the model.
- The model of care also facilitates patient goal attainment, provides more consistent care and encourages job satisfaction.

Conclusion

A key driver to the provision of quality care has been the development and implementation of different nursing models of care. This chapter began by describing the building blocks of nursing models of care and then went on to describe three important models of care that have been trialled in the care of older people: strengths-based care, person-centred care and the capabilities model of dementia care. This chapter has presented opportunities to reflect on practice as well as strategies through case scenarios showing how to implement some of the models of care. Strategies outlined that can influence a strengths-based approach to care include providing opportunities for patients to discuss the opportunities/skills they want to expand on and providing patients with opportunities to use the skills. Using the 10 capabilities to frame practice and care of people with dementia will support people with dementia to 'live a life worth living'.

Further reading

You may like to take a look at the following reading recommendations:

- The following reading provided by slide share – this slide presentation reviews staffing and nursing care delivery models. The slides were produced by Nidhin Mundackai: http://www.slideshare.net/nidhinmundackal/nursing-care-delivery
- The following reading from the Government of Western Australia Department of Health provides additional readings about models of care and service delivery models: http://www.agedcare.health.wa.gov.au/home/moc.cfm
- The final reading provides an overview of a strengths-based approach to care and evidence for its use: http://www.iriss.org.uk/resources/strengths-based-approaches-working-individuals

References

Aveyard, B. & Davies, S. (2006). Moving forward together: Evaluation of an action group involving staff and relatives within a nursing home for older people with dementia. *International Journal of Nursing Older People* 1(2), 95–104.

Brooker, D. (2007). *Person Centred Dementia Care: Making Services Better*. London: Jessica Kingsley Publications.

Butterworth, C. (2012). How to achieve a person-centred writing style in care plans. *Nursing Older People*, 24(8), 21–6.

Cooke, M., Moyle, W., Venturato, L., Walters, C. & Kinnane, J. (2013). Evaluation of an education intervention to implement a capability model of dementia. *Dementia: The International Journal of Social Research and Practice*. doi:10.1177/1471301213480158

Cox, A. (2001). BSW students favor strengths/empowerment based generalist practice. *Families in Society*, 82, 305–13.

Fast, B. & Chapin, R. (2000). *Strengths-based Care Management for Older Adults*. New York: Health Professions Press.

Feeley, N. & Gottlieb, N. (2000). Nursing approaches for working with family strengths and resources. *Journal of Family Nursing*, 6, 9–24.

Graybeal, C. (2001). Strengths-based social work assessment: Transforming the dominant paradigm. *Families in Society*, 82(3), 233–43.

Hooper, K. (2007). Rethinking social recovery in schizophrenia: What a capabilities approach might offer. *Social Science in Medicine*, 65(5), 868–79.

Jennings, B. (2000). A life greater than the sum of its sensations: Ethics, dementia, and the quality of life. In S. Albert and R. Logsdon (Eds.), *Assessing Quality of Life in Alzheimer's Disease*. New York: Springer,165–78.

King, I. (1997). King's theory of goal attainment in practice. *Nursing Science Quarterly*, 9(2), 61–6.

Kitwood, T. (1997). *Dementia Reconsidered*. Buckingham: Open University Press.

Moyle, W., Murfield, J., Venturato, L., Griffiths, S., Grimbeek, P., McAllister, M. & Marshall, J. (2013a). Dementia and its influence on quality of life and what it means to be valued: Family members' perceptions. *Dementia: The International Journal of Social Research and Practice*, 13(3), 412–25. doi: 10.1177/1471301212474147

Moyle, W., Venturato, L., Cooke, M., Hughes, J., van Wyk, S. & Marshall, J. (2013b). Promoting value in dementia care: Staff, resident and family experience of the capability model of dementia care. *Aging and Mental Health*, 17(5), 587–94. doi:10. 1080/13607863.2012.758233

Nolan, M., Brown, J., Davies, S., Nolan, J. & Keady, J. (2006). *The Senses Framework: Improving care for older people through a relationship-centred approach. Getting Research into Practice (GRiP) Report No. 2*. Sheffield, UK: University of Sheffield.

Nolan, M., Davies, S., Brown, J., Keady, J. & Nolan, J. (2004). Beyond person centred care: A new vision for gerontological nursing. *Journal of Clinical Nursing* 13 (s1), 45–53.

Nussbaum, M. (2000). *Women and Human Development: The Capabilities Approach*. New York: Cambridge University Press.

Nussbaum, M. (2004). *Hiding from Humanity*. Princeton: Princeton University Press.

Nussbaum, M. & Sen, A. (Eds.). (1993). *Quality of Life*. New York: Oxford University Press.

Orem, D. (1987). Orem's general theory of nursing. In R. Parse (Ed.), *Nursing Sciences: Major Paradigms, Theories and Critique*. Philadephia: W.B. Saunders.

Pearson, A., Vaughan, B. & Fitzgerald, M. (2005). *Nursing Models for Practice*. (3rd edition). Edinburgh: Butterworth Heinemann.

Rashid, T. & Ostermann, R. (2009). Strength-based assessment in clinical practice. *Journal of Clinical Psychology*, 65(5), 488–98.

Saleebey, D. (1996). The strengths perspective in social work practice: Extensions and cautions. *Social Work*, 41, 296–305.

Saleebey, D. (2000). Power in the people: Strengths and hope. *Advances in Social Work*, 1, 127–36.

Saleebey, D. (2002). *The Strengths Perspective in Social Work Practice*. (3rd edition). Boston: Allyn & Bacon.

Staudt, M., Howard, M.O. & Drake, B. (2001). The operationalization, implementation, and effectiveness of the strengths perspective: A review of empirical studies. *Journal of Social Service Research*, 27(3), 1–21.

Tresolini, C. & Pew-FetzerTask Force (1994). Health professions education and relationship-centred care. *Report of the Pew-Fetzer Task Force on Advancing Psychosocial Health Education.* San Francisco: Pew Health Professions Commission.

van den Pol-Grevelink, A., Jukema, J. & Smits, C. (2012). Person-centred care and job satisfaction of caregivers in nursing homes: A systematic review of the impact of different forms of person-centred care on various dimensions of job satisfaction. *International Journal of Geriatric Psychiatry,* 27, 219–29.

Nursing older people across aged care settings: interdisciplinary and intradisciplinary approaches

4

Marguerite Bramble

Learning objectives

After reading this chapter you will be able to:

1 Describe the paradigm shifts in aged care reform and their relevance to the strengths-based approach to care.

2 Outline the development of health care settings in the aged care system.

3 Describe the roles of the gerontological nurse as practice, advanced practice nurse, nurse practitioner, nurse educator and nurse manager.

4 Identify potential pathways when considering a profession in gerontology across aged care settings.

Introduction

Chapters 1 and 2 introduced the frameworks for nursing older people in the context of geriatric evaluation as a basis for strengths-based care across health care settings. Chapter 3 outlined the importance of nursing models in developing strengths-based care, with the aim to empower individual clients and their families, and improve quality of life. In this chapter the role of nurses in providing **case management** in **interdisciplinary** and **intradisciplinary** teams from **primary care** to palliative and end of life care will be discussed. Furthermore, the development of career pathways that provide opportunities for

Case management
An essential aspect of care delivery provided to individuals and including ongoing monitoring of support, detailed planning of clinical care and other aspects of delivery. Increases in intensity as need of clients become more complex.

student nurses to develop their skills, abilities and capabilities in gerontological nursing will be explored.

The paradigm shift in aged care

As discussed in Chapter 2 in Australia the wellness **paradigm** frames the aged care system and the design principles for the Living Longer, Living Better Aged Care Reform Package (Productivity Commission, 2011). In the 21st century aged care reform continues to shift the health focus from hospital-based to primary care services and improving integration between these areas. In New Zealand, as a result of the Health of Older People Strategy, services to this population have been developed across a variety of settings, including hospitals, primary health care services and other community health services (Hunter, 2012; Ramage, 2006). Whilst New Zealand's system of care is a little different from Australia's, the paradigm of developing primary health care as the entry point in the continuum of care for older people is similar (Australian Government Department of Health and Ageing, 2010; King, 2001).

Interdisciplinary
Involving the scope of two or more distinct disciplines.

Intradisciplinary
Occurring within the scope of a discipline, between people active in the discipline.

Primary care
First point of health care delivered in, and to, people living in their communities.

Primary health care is described as provision of access to comprehensive, community-based health care, including first point of call services for prevention, diagnosis and treatment of ill health, and ongoing management of chronic disease (Australian Government Department of Health and Ageing, 2010). Primary care includes a range of services provided by interdisciplinary teams of health professionals such as general practitioners, practice nurses, psychologists, physiotherapists, occupational therapists, nurse practitioners and community nurses.

Paradigm
A world view underlying the development of theories and models.

These teams work within the case management model of care to improve health outcomes for older people by using a preventive-based rather than an illness-based focus. This change in values and attitudes supports frameworks for strengths-based care (see Chapter 3).

Case management models of care

Case management models of care are successful in achieving early identification of complexity through the interdisciplinary approach to improve outcomes for older people. Using the case management approach, nurses in practice can coordinate teams to optimise client self-care, improve continuity of care across settings, enhance clients' quality of life, decrease length of hospitalisation, increase client and staff satisfaction, and promote cost-effective use of scarce re-sources (Hunter, 2012). Case management offers nurses an opportunity to demonstrate their roles as coordinators, managers and leaders in interdisciplinary health care teams with the aim to manage individual clients' health concerns. It is widely used internationally and in some countries, for example in the UK and the US, specialised nurses lead the case management of patients with stable chronic conditions such as diabetes and cardiovascular disease (Tabloski, 2010).

Case management and strengths-based care

The strengths-based approach to care, as discussed in Chapter 3, emphasises individual skills, capabilities and characteristics of clients by using the ROPES Model (Graybeal, 2001). This model (Chapter 3, pages 42–4) offers the opportunity for older people, their families and carers to not only understand their strengths but to mobilise them in partnership with nurses through case management. This approach to care promotes an integrated approach to the multi-dimensional needs of older people, as discussed in Chapters 1 and 2.

The aged care system and health settings

In Australia and New Zealand, and worldwide, aged care systems have been established to provide services targeted to the needs of older people and to provide them with opportunities to remain independent for as long as possible. This strategy is known as 'ageing in place'. Within the philosophy of ageing in place, care services are provided in various aged care settings (Figure 4.1) and will be discussed in the following sections.

Ageing in place

Worldwide the strategy of having people remain in their homes and communities for as long as possible avoids the costly option of institutional care and is therefore favoured by policy makers, health providers, and by many older people themselves (World Health Organization, 2007). In New Zealand the term 'ageing in place' relates to living in the community environment, with some level of independence, rather than in long-term care (Davey et al., 2004). In Australia ageing in place as a philosophy of care means that residents of a residential aged care facility (RACF) are able to remain in the same environment as their care needs increase (Commonwealth Department of Health and Age-ing, 2002). Ageing in place therefore is not merely about attachment to a par-ticular home; it is where the older person may continually transition within and between settings in the aged care system.

The strengths-based approach to care, as discussed in Chapter 3, enhances the meaning of ageing in place for older people as there is inherent understand-ing of the values and meaning of place and identity far beyond just that of home or housing (Feeley & Gottlieb, 2000). More importantly it relates to maintaining a sense of identity both through independence and autonomy and through caring relationships and roles in the places where people live (Wiles et al., 2011).

Consumer directed care
Described as both a philosophy and an orientation to a service delivery option where consumers control and choose the services they get, including what, when, how, where and who provides those services.

Figure 4.1 provides a summary of the range of services avail-able to older clients transitioning across the continuum from pri-mary care to end of life care. Current aged care reforms in the 21st century aim to build an integrated system of care that of-fers more choice and control for older people. They also have a greater emphasis on **consumer directed care** as older people

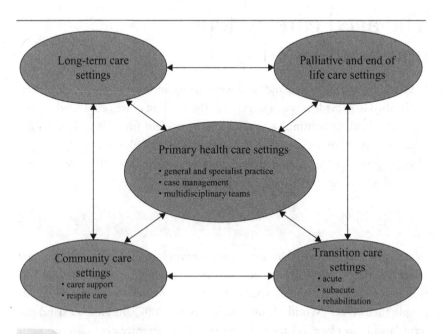

FIGURE
4.1
The aged care system and health care settings

transition across settings within the care continuum. These transitions may occur over a number of weeks, months or years and are reflective of an individual's journey through ageing, or ageing in place. The types of care and health care settings older people may encounter in this journey are outlined in the following sections.

Types of care in the aged care system

As discussed in Chapters 2 and 10 the ageing population requires a number of different types of care to achieve equity of access and to cater for individual needs of clients and families. In Australia services range across settings from Respite Care and Home Care Packages that support clients and families in their homes to long-term care in RACFs. Residents in RACFs are classified as high or low care based on their Aged Care Funding Instrument (ACFI) appraisal and may access extra services as of 30 June 2014, with the introduction of Consumer Directed Care Packages (Australian Government Department of Health and Ageing, 2014). These types of care and settings in which they are provided will be discussed in the following sections.

The primary health care settings

Primary health care settings are developing to ensure that people can access the health care they need, when they need it, where they need it. This helps people better manage their own health and plays an important role in preventing disease. In Australia the implementation of this new single entry to aged care services is linked to other health reforms such as the **local hospital networks, Medicare Local Programs** and **Transition Care Programs**, which increase service accessibility and concurrently aim to build a skilled practice and aged care nursing workforce (Australian Government Department of Health and Ageing, 2011).

The community care settings

As befits the strengths-based approach (see Chapter 3) an increasing range of home or community based services are being provided to encourage autonomy and independence for older

Local hospital networks Small groups of local hospitals, or an individual hospital, linking services within a region or through specialist networks across a state or territory.

Medicare Local Program(s) Primary health care practices that coordinate and deliver services based on community need, including after-hours GP services, immunisation, mental health support, targeted and tailored services for those in need, and e-health.

Transition Care Programs Programs for older people who have been in hospital but need more help to recover and time to make a decision about the best place for them to live in the longer term.

Multidisciplinary team Composed of members from more than one discipline so that the team can offer a greater breadth of services to patients.

people in their home environment. These services range from domestic support and personal care provided by formal carers to increased level of support such as Community Aged Care Packages (CACPs), Extended Aged Care at Home (EACH) Packages and Extended Aged Care at Home Dementia (EACHD) Packages (Australian Government Department of Health and Ageing, 2013). These home care service packages also involve the **multidisciplinary team**, such as nurses, physiotherapists, occupational therapists, podiatrists and social workers. Nurses are often responsible for coordinating geriatric assessment and case management of these packages of services for individuals and families. Implicit in this role is to ensure that people receive the most culturally appropriate and cost-effective services suited to their complex needs within the context of chronic conditions. The case management approach also reduces the need for emergency and hospital care by better managing chronic conditions in partnership with clients (Tabloski, 2010).

Transitional care settings

Depending on their functional and health status some older people make multiple transitions across acute care, **subacute care** and respite care in

Subacute care Provides assessment and rehabilitation for complex conditions following or preceding acute care admission. Usually for a maximum of three months.

RACF settings, with increasing risk of problems with medications, miscommunication and adverse events (Australian Government Department of Health and Ageing, 2011). The main aim of Transition Care Programs therefore is to facilitate and coordinate continuity of care across health and aged care settings. As identified in Figure 4.1 this may be between primary and community, acute care, subacute and RACF settings. As Transition Care Programs become more established across health care settings, models of care based on integration between health care settings, such as the strengths-based model, will provide more equity across the care continuum (see Chapter 3).

Acute care settings

Although **acute care settings** are important in providing appropriate services to older people according to need, the strategy is to reduce hospital stays and provide more targeted services and specialised care in primary, subacute, transitional and **long-term care settings**. In hospitals there has also been the development of specialised units such as geriatric acute care units, rehabilitation units, acute care for elderly people (ACE) units for people with dementia, transitional care units (TCUs), aged care service emergency teams (ASETs), outpatient clinics and Hospital at Home models of care (Hunter, 2012). Some of these units are developed within the Subacute and Transition Care Programs.

> **Acute care settings** Settings that provide short-term medical treatment, usually in a hospital, for patients having an acute illness or injury or recovering from surgery.
>
> **Long-term care settings** Residential care for individuals above the age of 65 or with a chronic or disabling condition that needs constant supervision.

Subacute care settings

Subacute care settings provide care to older clients for up to three months and may include rehabilitation, geriatric evaluation and case management. Some subacute services are colloquially referred to as low dependency or step up and step down care, meaning that care can either precede (and potentially avert) a hospital admission or follow an acute hospital admission. Most subacute services can be provided on either an inpatient or ambulatory basis. Care is goal oriented and interventions are aimed at assessing and managing often complex conditions by multidisciplinary teams to maximise independence and quality of life for people with disabling conditions (State Government of Victoria Department of Health, 2003).

Long-term care settings

Institutions providing long-term care in Australia are called residential aged care facilities (RACFs) and in New Zealand these institutions are called 'rest homes'. Transition to RACFs or rest homes is a pivotal point of ageing in place as people make the major and permanent move from their homes to reside in long-term care. Older people residing in long-term care are therefore termed 'residents', and as such have additional legal rights and protection in their new home environment. As discussed in Chapter 3 the philosophy of strengths-based nursing in long-term care provides the basis for the implementation of new models of care to improve quality of life and individualised care for clients.

Nursing care provided in long-term care settings ranges from supervision of direct care activities such as activities of daily living (ADLs) to complex, palliative and end of life care (see Chapters 10 to 13). As the functional capacity of a resident declines and more complex care is required nurses manage individual residents' transition to more complex and clinically based care, ideally within the long-term care, rather than acute care setting. Newer models of strengths-based care and advanced practice in case management will involve nurses fostering a team-based approach when supervising **endorsed enrolled nurses** (EENs) and direct care staff in residential care. It will also mean assuming clinical management, supervisory, leadership and consultative roles in providing best practice, evidence-based care to clients and families.

> **Endorsed enrolled nurses** Second level nurses who provide nursing care, working under the direction and supervision of registered nurses. Have endorsement to administer medications.

In response to cultural diversity in Australia and New Zealand some long-term care facilities target their services to culturally and linguistically diverse (CALD) and indigenous populations as well as gay and lesbian groups, and specific religious-based communities. In rural and remote areas long-term care facilities link to government, community and specialist medical services through e-health to provide the best outcomes for their clients (Australian Government Department of Health and Ageing, 2010). A growing area of need in long-term care is palliative and end of life care, which will be further discussed in Chapters 10 to 13.

The role of the gerontological nurse across health care settings

As discussed in Chapter 1 knowledge about the ageing process and risk factors associated with physical, cognitive and psychosocial changes is required by all nurses caring for older adults (Hunter, 2012). As the **aged care system** continues to evolve to meet the needs of ageing populations, opportunities will increase for gerontological nurses to assume more responsibility for coordination of services in interdisciplinary teams across a number of health care settings. Strong intradisciplinary linkages between nurse educators, managers, researchers and practice nurses will also be vital to ensure relevant education and models of care form the basis for role development for all nurses, from students to advanced nurse clinicians, managers and leaders in practice. Across the continuum of learning these emerging roles, or pathways, take shape from a student nurse's first clinical placement in a health care setting and provide the foundations for continuous learning and career development within the professional scope and ethical standards

> **Aged care system** Provides the framework for older people to have timely access to appropriate care and support services.

of nursing practice. These roles range from **client advocate** to nurse practitioner and the key aspects of each role are identified in Table 4.1 (Tabloski, 2010; Touhy & Jett, 2012). The following sections discuss in more detail career pathways in which these roles can be supported and formalised.

Client advocate
Someone who advances the rights of older persons and educates others regarding negative stereotypes of ageing.

TABLE 4.1 *Nursing roles in the continuum of learning*

NURSING ROLE	DESCRIPTION
Nurse advocate	Advances the rights of older persons and educates others regarding negative stereotypes of ageing.
Nurse educator	Provides information and instructions about healthy ageing, disease detection, treatment of disease and rehabilitation for older people and their families.
Practice/clinical manager	Maintains current relevant information regarding government regulations and reforms. Provides nursing leadership in a variety of health care settings.
Practice/clinical consultant	Consults with and advises others who are providing nursing care to older patients with complex health care problems. Participates in the development of clinical pathways and quality assurance standards and implementation of evidence-based practice.
Clinical /academic researcher	Collaborates with clinicians and other researchers to develop clinically based studies and models of care. Communicates relevant research findings to others, and participates in the presentation of findings at gerontological conferences and publications.
Advanced practice nurse/nurse practitioner	Registered nurses who have acquired the expert knowledge base as a result of advanced education, complex decision making skills and clinical competencies for expanded practice (minimum of five years clinical practice).

Source: Adapted from Tabloski, 2010, p. 36

Potential pathways for the gerontological nursing profession

For student, novice and experienced nurses, having clear career pathways and recognition systems supports professional development, job satisfaction and can inspire retention by opening doors within health that previously may not have been a considered option (Heath, 2002). With the implementation of reform in the aged care system, building more formal professional development pathways would also build nurses' understanding of how current best practice protocols may be integrated into settings across the continuum in cost-effective and care-efficient ways. Future directions for intradisciplinary nursing teams include developing the role of practice nurses in case management, interprofessional communication, ageing in place and development of models for end of life care in the home and long-term residential care (Touhy & Jett, 2012).

Scope of practice

As discussed in Chapter 1 the scope of the gerontological nurse is to ensure comprehensive geriatric needs evaluation is provided to fully assess the complex needs of older clients. Nursing students build understanding of the profession's scope of practice from their first year of study, with the aim to attain the knowledge, skills and attitudes to be competent as a graduate registered nurse (RN). The scope of professional practice includes professional standards such as competency standards, codes of ethics, conduct and practice and public need, demand and expectation (Nursing and Midwifery Board of Australia, 2007).

Once a student of nursing achieves the profession's competency standards and graduates as an RN in the nursing profession, pathways should be available to build expertise and specialisation in gerontological nursing. In Australia and New Zealand further pathways are developing through formal recognition of the scope of practice for practice nurses, advanced practice nurses, nurse consultants and nurse practitioners. Recent major developments in these roles will be discussed in the following sections.

Developing practice nurses in general practice

The aim of the Nursing in General Practice Program (NiGP) in Australia is to support and build the capacity of the nursing workforce in this area and to build the capacity of Medicare Locals to provide primary health care services. There is a growing emphasis on the value of the nursing role in primary health care, including multidisciplinary and collaborative care (Australian Government Department of Health and Ageing, 2011). The program will be implemented across each state and territory and will include online and face-to-face conferences, postgraduate and other professional development opportunities which support beginning and advanced practice nurses, Aboriginal health workers and nurse practitioners in general practice (Australian Government Department of Health and Ageing, 2011).

Developing practice nurses in rural and remote areas

In Australia, it is often rural areas that are most in need of health care for older people and nurses provide a pivotal role in its delivery (Australian Government Department of Health and Ageing, 2011). Medicare rebates are now available in **e-health** eligible areas, and in eligible RACFs and Aboriginal medical services throughout Australia, for clinical services provided by a nurse as the health professional located with the patient during the video consultation (Australian Government Department of Health and Ageing, 2011). In this situation, the nurse would be present in a regional, rural or remote area with the older person receiving care, and the medical specialist would be located elsewhere, usually in a metropolitan area.

> **E-health**
> A system that enables a personally controlled, secure online summary of a client's health information.

Developing the nurse case manager

Across aged care settings there are increased opportunities for case management roles for nurses working in interdisciplinary teams to achieve holistic assessment and management. Similarly new health paradigms are seeing the evolution of leadership roles for nurses as case managers. This role ranges from assessing primary care health status, quality of life and effectiveness of health care to establishing collaborative partnerships in multidisciplinary service settings, which may be electronically linked (Cohen & Cesta, 2005). Case management is increasingly seen as the most cost effective delivery of services, as a way of delivering quality care and providing to individual client needs (Cohen & Cesta, 2005).

The advanced practice nurse and nurse practitioner

The role of aged care nurse practitioners (NPs) is well recognised internationally, including New Zealand, but in Australia is still in its infancy (Lee, 2009). As a clinical career path for nurses, the advanced practice nursing (APN) role was introduced in 1986 with the subsequent introduction of the clinical nurse specialist and clinical nurse consultant roles. The NP role developed a decade later to further expand the APN role. The scope of practice of the NP is determined by the context in which the NP is authorised to practise (Nursing and Midwifery Board of Australia, 2013). For example an NP practising in a long-term care setting would target interventions and measure outcomes based on the needs of that group of clients (Lee, 2009). Current research shows that NPs in aged care can deliver effective outcomes in the areas of dementia and delirium management and medication management (Borbasi et al., 2010; Burge et al., 2010).

Generally NP roles have emerged in response to the need for new models of service delivery and improved interventions that are more responsive to diversity of need. The International Council of Nurses (ICN) defines the role of APNs as RNs who have acquired the expert knowledge base as a result of advanced education, complex decision making skills and clinical competencies for expanded practice.

In Australia the NP is an RN, educated to function autonomously and collaboratively in an advanced and expanded clinical nursing role (Australian Government, 2010). The role includes assessment and management of clients and may include: the direct referral of clients to other health care professionals, prescribing medications and ordering diagnostic investigations. In New Zealand NPs have additional scope as RNs by having access to provider numbers, case managing clients with highly complex chronic conditions, assisting clients to access services, diagnosing, treating and monitoring chronic diseases (Lee, 2009).

Practice and curriculum development pathways

In Australia and New Zealand roles and career pathways for gerontological nurses are developing rapidly in response to the need for increased clinical expertise and advanced, complex decision making skills across health care settings. Figure 4.2 provides an overview of the links between practice and curriculum pathways of development. These pathways are useful to provide guidance for nurses in considering a career in gerontological nursing.

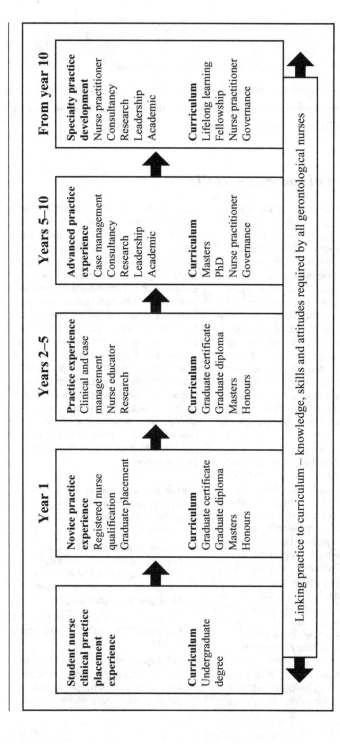

Student nurse clinical practice placement experience	Novice practice experience Registered nurse qualification Graduate placement	Practice experience Clinical and case management Nurse educator Research	Advanced practice experience Case management Consultancy Research Leadership Academic	Specialty practice development Nurse practitioner Consultancy Research Leadership Academic
	Year 1	Years 2–5	Years 5–10	From year 10
Curriculum Undergraduate degree	Curriculum Graduate certificate Graduate diploma Masters Honours	Curriculum Graduate certificate Graduate diploma Masters Honours	Curriculum Masters PhD Nurse practitioner Governance	Curriculum Lifelong learning Fellowship Nurse practitioner Governance

Linking practice to curriculum – knowledge, skills and attitudes required by all gerontological nurses

FIGURE
4.2   *Practice and curriculum development pathways*

Professional development in the context of ageing

The following scenario is based on a real life situation and exemplifies the benefits for students and novice nurses to reflect on their abilities as well as their knowledge, skills and attitudes in planning a career pathway.

Professional development – Jodie

Case scenario 4.1

Jodie is 23 years old and graduated with her Bachelor of Nursing degree two years ago. During her student years she worked as a formal carer in a RACF to top up her income and she often spoke of how she initially 'hated it'. However it wasn't long before she discovered she had a natural ability with older people and particularly those residents with dementia. She decided working in an RACF or similar setting was the 'only place' she wanted to be. This decision was also influenced by her student experiences in other clinical placements, where she found her commitment to providing person-centred care was not acknowledged or supported.

Following graduation Jodie first worked in a dementia secure unit for her graduate year where she extended her skills and knowledge of person-centred care. She then began working in a subacute care geriatric unit attached to a cosmopolitan hospital where she felt inspired by the person-centred approach of the geriatrician and the multidisciplinary team.

However, two years since graduation, Jodie has been feeling that professional development opportunities to build her scope as an RN are not enough to support her emerging abilities as a nurse leader in practice. With support from her mentors she has since launched herself on a career pathway, which will help her achieve an ambition to be a leader in aged care

nursing, specialising in psychogeriatric dementia care. She has commenced a Graduate Certificate in Ageing and Dementia, which she believes will provide her with the evidence-based knowledge for 'honing practice' and continuous improvement in this clinical area. When she has completed her Masters' qualification and the required five years practice in psychogeriatric care, Jodie then aims to commence a specialty clinical Masters in Mental Health Nursing which will give her the qualifications for nurse practitioner registration and competency to work 'autonomously as a leader'. Jodie has chosen both academic and clinical practice leaders to provide her with the right mix to support her professional career pathway.

Reflective questions
Read and reflect on the case example of Jodie and address the following questions:

> In your experience in clinical placement have you identified areas of natural ability in relation to knowledge, skills and attitudes to older people in your care?

> Where do you see yourself one year/ five years/10 years from graduation as an RN?

> Are there particular areas of interest in gerontology that may develop for you as a basis for professional development and a career pathway?

he nurse's role as client advocate

Case scenario 4.2

Joan Blue is aged 75 and has lived alone since the death of her husband eight years ago. She has not had any community or home care support as she is very resistant to accepting care from others outside her family. She has one daughter who is concerned that her living situation is deteriorating and osteoporosis is causing increasing frailty.

Joan was taken to hospital following a recent fall in the street and sustained a fractured right wrist and femur. Following surgery and rehabilitation she was transferred to the transitional care unit for assessment as she has become dependent on others for dressing, meal preparation and bathing.

You are completing your three month placement as a graduate registered nurse in the transitional unit. While caring for Joan she confides in you that she is concerned about her daughter's refusal to consider any other option for her but long-term care in an RACF. A family case conference with the multidisciplinary team has been organised for later in the week to discuss strategies for Joan's future but she feels she has not been included in these discussions. You have decided that Joan needs a client advocate who can discuss her situation with her daughter and provide more decision making. You approach your clinical mentor to discuss the client advocate role further.

You review Joan's geriatric evaluation using the strengths-based approach and ROPES Assessment. You note that communication between Joan and her daughter has deteriorated over the years and her daughter has not considered her mother's overall needs and rights in making decisions about her future.

Reflective questions

Read and reflect on the case example of Joan and reflect on the following questions:

> In your role as client advocate for Joan what are the main issues you would consider with your clinical mentor?

> Who are the members of the multidisciplinary team you would most likely approach prior to the family conference?

> What other options would there be for Joan at this stage other than moving to an RACF?

Summary

- Health care reform continues to shift the focus of care of older adults to new models of nursing care such as the strengths-based approach.
- Health care settings in the aged care system are described as primary, community, acute, subacute and long-term residential aged care.
- Improvements to the aged care system and client service provision bring with them advanced practice and leadership opportunities for gerontological nurses.
- Professional development and career pathways are required to advance these opportunities for nurses.

Conclusion

This chapter has examined aged care reform and the healthy ageing and ageing in place paradigms. New models of service provision such as the strengths-based approach and case management offer opportunities for professional development and career pathways for nurses in this exciting era of health care. Nurses can make a major contribution to best practice care as clinicians, managers, researchers and educators in advanced practice and leadership roles.

Further reading

You may like to take a look at the following reading recommendations:

- My Aged Care website for further information on standards in long-term care: http://www.myagedcare.gov.au/accreditation-standards-0
- For information on standards and packages in community care in Australia refer to Australian Government Department of Health and Ageing website: http://www.livinglongerlivingbetter.gov.au/internet/living/publishing.nsf/Content/home-care-packages-program-guidelines
- Australia's Department of Health: http://www.health.gov.au/
- Australian Institute of Health and Welfare: http://www.aihw.gov.au/

References

Australian Government. (2010). *National Health (Collaborative Arrangements for Nurse Practitioners). Determination 2010: ComLaw*. Canberra.

Australian Government Department of Health and Ageing. (2010). *Building a 21st Century Primary Health Care System: Australia's First National Primary Health Care Strategy*. Canberra.

Australian Government Department of Health and Ageing. (2011). *National Health Reform*. Retrieved from http://www.yourhealth.gov.au/internet/yourhealth/publishing.nsf/content/medilocals

Australian Government Department of Health and Ageing. (2013). *Home Care Packages Program Guidelines – August 2013*. Retrieved from http://www.livinglongerlivingbetter.gov.au/internet/living/publishing.nsf/Content/home-care-packages-program-guidelines

Australian Government Department of Health and Ageing. (2014). *Detailed Questions and Answers: Residential Care.* Retrieved from http://www. livinglongerlivingbetter.gov.au/internet/living/publishing.nsf/Content/ageing-legislative-questions-and-answers-toc~ageing-legislative-questions-and-answers-residential top

Borbasi, S., Emmanuel, E., Farrelly, B. & Ashcroft, J. (2010). A nurse practitioner initiated model of service delivery in caring for people with dementia. *Contemporary Nurse: A Journal for the Australian Nursing Profession,* 1(2), 49–60.

Burge, D., Kent, W., Verdon, J., Voogt, S. & Haines, H. (2010). Nurse practitioners are well placed to lead in the effective management of delirium. *Australian Journal of Advanced Nursing* 28(1), 67–73.

Cohen, E. & Cesta, T. (2005). *Nursing Case Management: From Essentials to Advanced Practice Applications.* (4th edition). St Louis: Elsevier Mosby.

Commonwealth Department of Health and Ageing. (2002). *Ageing in Place: A Guide for Providers of Residential Aged Care.* Canberra.

Davey, J., Nana, G., de Joux, V. & Arcus, M. (2004). *Accommodation Options for Older People in Aotearoa/New Zealand.* Wellington: NZ Institute for Research on Ageing/Business & Economic Research Ltd, Centre for Housing Research Aotearoa/New Zealand.

Feeley, N. & Gottlieb, N. (2000). Nursing approaches for working with family strengths and resources. *Journal of Family Nursing,* 6, 9–24.

Graybeal, C. (2001). Strengths-based social work assessment: Transforming the dominant paradigm. *Families in Society,* 82(3), 233–43.

Heath, P. (2002). *National Review of Nursing Education: Our Duty of Care.* Canberra: Commonwealth of Australia.

Hunter, S. (2012). *Miller's Nursing for Wellness in Older Adults.* Philadelphia: Wolters Kluwer/Lippincott Williams & Wilkins.

King, A. (2001). *The Primary Health Care Strategy.* Retrieved from http://www.moh. govt.nz

Lee, C. (2009). *Role of the Gerontological Nurse Practitioner in Australia.* (Doctor of Philosophy). Adelaide: University of Adelaide.

Nursing and Midwifery Board of Australia. (2007). *A National Framework for the Development of Decision-making Tools for Nursing and Midwifery Practice.* Melbourne.

Nursing and Midwifery Board of Australia. (2013). *Competency Standards of the Nurse Practitioner.* Melbourne.

Productivity Commission. (2011). *Caring for Older Australians.* Canberra: Australian Government.

Ramage, C. (2006). *Evaluation of Strategies for Ageing in Place.* Auckland: The University of Auckland.

State Government of Victoria Department of Health. (2003). *Victorian Government Health Information: Sub-acute Care Services*. Retrieved from http://www.health.vic.gov.au/subacute/

Tabloski, P. (2010). *Gerontological Nursing* (2nd edition). New Jersey: Pearson.

Touhy, T. & Jett, K. (2012). *Ebersole & Hess' Toward Healthy Ageing: Human Needs & Nursing Response*: St Louis: Elsevier.

Wiles, J., Leibing, A., Guberman, N., Reeve, J. & Allen, R. (2011). The meaning of 'Ageing in Place' to older people. *The Gerontologist*. doi: 10.1093/geront/gnr098

World Health Organization (WHO). (2007). *Global Age-friendly Cities Project*. Geneva.

Evidence-based nursing interventions in primary care: a strengths-based approach

5

Marguerite Bramble

Learning objectives

After reading this chapter you will be able to:

1. Have an understanding of the development of evidence-based primary care in Australia and New Zealand.

2. Outline the types of evidence-based nursing interventions that promote health and wellness for older adults in primary care.

3. Discuss how to use the strengths-based approach in primary care.

4. Demonstrate understanding of professional development opportunities for nurses in primary care.

Introduction

This chapter will discuss the development of current and future evidence-based nursing interventions that promote **health** and **wellness** in the provision of primary clinical care for older people. As outlined in Chapters 1 and 2 older people, particularly those described as the old-old (85 years and over), are increasingly susceptible to multiple physiological changes of ageing and chronic illness. Chapter 3 examined nursing care models that guide practice and the development of strengths-based, person-centred, relationship-centred and the Capabilities Model of Dementia Care to support the health and well-being of older people. This chapter

Health The ability of older adults to function at their highest capacity despite the presence of age related changes and risk factors.

Wellness Outcome (or positive functional consequence) for older adults whose well-being and quality of life is improved through nursing interventions.

builds on Chapter 4, which introduced the primary health care setting as the first point of access to multidisciplinary, community-based health care, including first point of call services to provide continuity of care.

The role of the gerontological nurse in primary care

Primary care
First point of health care delivered in, and to, people living in their communities.

Health promotion interventions
Interventions that focus on behaviour changes, including disease prevention and health maintenance.

Curative
Health care traditionally oriented towards seeking a cure for an existent disease or medical condition.

Rehabilitation
A treatment or treatments designed to facilitate the process of recovery from injury, illness or disease to as normal a condition as possible.

Self-efficacy
The ability of the person to regulate their motivation, thought processes and emotional states, and appropriate behavioural changes. Self-efficacy affects the older person's functional status during rehabilitation.

In community-based **primary care** the role of the gerontological nurse is to establish relationships with older people in order to provide 'first point of call', comprehensive geriatric evaluation and holistic care based on an individual client's needs. As discussed in Chapter 3 relationship-centred care focuses on the multidimensional needs of older people by building important relationships with them and health professionals across health care settings as an imperative to optimise care. This approach to nursing practice is reflected in a Scottish definition of gerontological nursing:

[a] relationship centred approach that promotes healthy ageing and the achievement of well-being in the older person and their family carers, enabling them to adapt to the older person's health and life changes and to face ongoing life challenges. (Kelly et al., 2005, p. 19)

As discussed in Chapter 4, when establishing relationships with clients in primary care settings, nurses develop case management strategies that aim to actively involve older people in their health and well-being and motivate behaviour change through **health promotion interventions**. In addition to skills that enable older people to optimise health and well-being, gerontological nurses require knowledge of **curative** and **rehabilitation** aspects of care. These aspects facilitate **self-efficacy** and enable a strengths-based approach to chronic and long-term conditions, as well as palliative and end of life care (Tolson, Booth & Schofield, 2011a). Models of palliative and end of life care are further discussed in Chapters 10 to 13.

The development of primary care

Worldwide, models of primary care have developed in response to the increasing costs of caring for an ageing population, the associated increase in chronic disease and the inadequacies of acute care systems in providing appropriate holistic care for older people (Bodenheimer, Wagner & Grumbach, 2002). The World Health Organization defines primary health care as incorporating curative treatment given by the first contact provider along with promotional, preventive and rehabilitative services provided by multidisciplinary teams of health care professionals working collaboratively (World Health Organization, 2008). Recent reviews have shown that the strength of a country's primary care system is associated with improved population health outcomes for all, higher patient or client satisfaction, and reduced overall health care spending (Australian Government Department of Health and Ageing, 2010). This includes improving access and equity to primary health care services for all cultures and socioeconomic groups within societies.

In Australia and New Zealand health and aged care systems continue to improve their economic and funding arrangements with the aim to provide best practice care. As discussed in Chapter 4, in primary care there is a call to re-evaluate the role of the professional nurse and the types of nurses that will be needed in practice (Tolson, Booth & Schofield, 2011b). New Zealand's Primary Health Care Strategy, which has been implemented through the district health boards, has identified that for primary care to be successful it needs to be socially acceptable and scientifically sound first level care provided by a suitably trained nursing and health professional workforce (King, 2001). Similarly in Australia health reform is well under way in the primary community sector through the **Medicare Local Program** (Australian Government Department of Health and Ageing, 2010). Both of these programs have a focus on developing nursing capability in general practice clinics as the first point of call to provide holistic assessment for clients. As discussed in Chapter 4 nurses have the opportunity to play a significant leadership role in building success in these areas through the development of case management models of care using evidence-based practice interventions.

Medicare Local Program(s) Primary health care practices that coordinate and deliver services based on community need, including after-hours GP services, immunisation, mental health support, targeted and tailored services for those in need, and e-health.

Understanding evidence-based practice

Evidence-based practice is the cornerstone for providing scientifically sound, safe and effective care by all health professionals involved in the care of older people. Initially the scientific parameters of evidence-based practice developed in medicine, with the establishment of the **Cochrane Collaboration** and the Cochrane Collection Database. Although a number of primary care evidence-based nursing interventions reside in the Cochrane Collection (Gillespie et al., 2009), the Joanna Briggs Institute (JBI) is the home of most evidence-based nursing interventions (Chenoworth, 2010). Within the institute, the Joanna Briggs Aged Care Unit and the Care Quality Association (ACQA) develop nursing standards in practice in aged care that are built on the best available evidence (Joanna Briggs Institute, 2011). In Australia policy practice links are also developing in the primary care sector through the development of age friendly principles that support evidence-based care focused on improving quality of life for older people (Australian Health Ministers' Advisory Council, 2004; Menec & Nowicki, 2014). The development of nursing interventions that support quality of life are further discussed in Chapter 9.

Evidence-based practice The practice of health care in which the practitioner systematically finds, appraises and uses the most current and valid research findings as the basis for clinical decisions.

Cochrane Collaboration An independent non-profit organisation consisting of a group of more than 31 000 volunteers in more than 120 countries. The collaboration was formed to organise medical research information in a systematic way in the interests of evidence-based medicine.

Evidence-based interventions in nursing practice

Evidence-based nursing practice is conceptualised by the JBI Model of Evidence-Based Healthcare as **clinical decision making** that considers (1) the best available current evidence; (2) the context in which the care is delivered; (3) client preference and (4) the professional judgement of the health professional (Pearson, Weeks & Stern, 2010). Within this framework major sources of evidence available to nurses in practice from the JBI database are not only scientifically or quantitatively based, but also qualitative or experiential, so that client and person-centred measures of appropriateness and meaningfulness can be used to influence nursing decisions (Pearson, Weeks & Stern, 2010).

In this person-centred framework research evidence provides an evidence-based framework for nurses to make clinical decisions with clients based on their individual needs (Pearson, Weeks & Stern, 2010). This means that not only do nurses base their care on clinical expertise and the latest evidence, they can also take a 'marketing approach' to decision making, whereby nurses orientate their care to the client and carer experience, and to their expectations of care, as well as responding to an individual's clinical signs and symptoms and life stage (Tolson, Booth & Schofield, 2011a). As case managers and coordinators of care it is important in this context for gerontological nurses to make the connection between relevant theory, evidence, values, relational care and changes of ageing to deliver safe and effective care (Tolson, Booth & Schofield, 2011a).

> **Clinical decision making** A balance of experience, awareness, knowledge and information gathering, using appropriate assessment tools, colleagues and evidence based practice as guidance.

As outlined in the strengths-based approach presented in Chapter 3, a person-centred framework establishes the platform for nurses to achieve continuous improvement in providing the best outcomes for clients and families based on their values, preferences and experiences (Booth et al., 2011). When implementing values-based models of care such as those discussed in Chapter 3, nurses in practice also need to ensure that individual client rights are preserved through adherence to the Code of Professional Conduct for Nurses (Nursing and Midwifery Board of Australia, 2011; Tolson, Booth & Schofield, 2011a).

In Australia and New Zealand the development of evidence-based nursing interventions for older people based on models of care that are relationship-centred and appropriate to the primary care context is in its infancy. The following section presents a model currently under development in Australia.

The development of an Australian evidence-based primary care model

Across Australia the primary health sector is under reform through the development of 61 Medicare Locals, which have been established to fund new models of community services in localised urban and rural areas. These reforms aim to develop new primary care nursing and medical models, in collaboration with allied health professionals, to provide holistic patient care. A major role of the Australian Medicare Local Alliance (AML Alliance) is to provide leadership and coordination for Medicare Locals to support and build nursing capability in general practice. More nurses will be required to fulfil the role of the community, practice and advanced practice nurse, including providing: (1) preventive care, such as immunisation; (2) screening such as Pap smears; (3) lifestyle education and health promotion and (4) clinical activities, such as wound assessments, nurse clinics, community home visits, coordination of care for patients with chronic conditions, emergency care and triage (Australian Government Department of Health and Ageing, 2010).

Within this model it is envisaged that the number of nurse practitioners will also increase in primary care to provide services to older people. Nurse practitioners will have the capability to conduct routine annual comprehensive health assessments, which are available for all older people 75 years and over, followed by nursing diagnosis, care planning and referral to other health professionals where indicated (Australian Government Department of Health and Ageing, 2010). The primary health nurse practitioner will also provide additional expertise in chronic condition management and experience in care coordination, as well as prescribing medications, ordering pathology and X-rays and referring to other health professionals.

An area of priority for the AML Alliance is to build primary care nursing sustainability by developing age friendly services. An example of this is the evidence-based age friendly program that has been developed in emergency departments in Australia and is discussed in detail in Chapter 9. Achieving sustainability will also rely on nurses advancing their practice roles in primary care by drawing on credible evidence and optimising outcomes based on sound clinical decisions about resource allocation, nursing interventions and client assessments through evidence-based person-centred practice (Chenoworth, 2010). An example of a new model of practice is presented in the reflective activity.

Reflective activity: a multidisciplinary model in primary care

An innovative multidisciplinary model of care coordination and chronic disease case management is currently being trialled in a rural general practice in Australia. The model aims to reduce the number of admissions to acute care by focusing on promoting good health, early intervention and better management of chronic disease in the community. To achieve the goals of the National Primary Health Care Strategy the model has the following characteristics:

- The general practice has the services of a nurse practitioner (NP) with expertise in chronic condition management and experience in case management.
- The NP coordinates the completion of comprehensive health assessments for all new patients and annually for those over 75 years, with an additional focus on the 40–49 year old group where preventive care and lifestyle behaviour counselling regarding risk factors can be particularly effective.
- From health assessments, follow up planning and care is provided jointly by the general practitioner (GP) and NP with a focus on chronic disease management. Gaps in care are identified and either acted on by the NP or referred to the GP or allied health professionals.
- The model supports professional development opportunities for practice nurses by working within a multidisciplinary team to provide holistic health care. Professional development and training is also focused on care that provides evidence-based chronic disease management and care coordination.
- All staff are also trained in using the chronic disease management care planning tool cdmNet, which is a systematic database that allows sharing of clinical information electronically between health providers and manages Medicare compliance.
- The practice nurse is also trained in health promotion, motivational interviewing and setting individual goals with clients to support lifestyle behaviour change.
- Data collection focuses on patient outcomes in relation to reduced hospitalisation for older people with chronic disease, mainly chronic obstructive pulmonary disease, pneumonia, diabetes, heart disease and dementia (Australian Government Department of Health and Ageing, 2010).

You are a newly graduated nurse and you have just commenced your clinical placement as part of the team in this general practice clinic under the mentorship of the practice nurse. Consider:

- What other areas of training and professional development would you need to provide care within the strengths-based approach?
- How would you best use available clinical evidence-based guidelines to build your expertise in person-centred care?
- How would you best use available clinical evidence-based guidelines to build your expertise in care coordination and case management?

An evidence-based primary assessment model in New Zealand

As part of its Positive Ageing Strategy and Health of Older People Strategy, the New Zealand Ministry of Health developed evidence-based recommendations for appropriate and effective assessment processes to identify personal, social, functional and clinical needs of people over the age of 65 years. A major recommendation of the strategy was that the evidence-based interRAI-Minimum Data Set for Home Care be used for the comprehensive assessment of older people in New Zealand. The interRAI-Minimum Data Set for Home Care overview and the EASY-Care instrument are also recommended for **screening and proactive assessments** (New Zealand Guidelines Group, 2003, pp. 25–6). In this primary health promotion model distinctions are drawn between screening assessment, proactive assessment, comprehensive assessment and carer assessment. The aims of these forms of assessment are to improve outcomes for those in the community and their carers most at risk of developing chronic diseases and functional impairment. However the model has limitations in encouraging and empowering clients to change their own behaviour, as described in the strengths-based approach.

> **Screening and proactive assessments** Detect problems and identify potential for multidimensional health or functional impairment at an early stage in order to initiate interventions designed to improve health, for example, diabetes, depression.

Using the strengths-based approach in health promotion

When using the strengths-based approach, promoting health in later life means understanding the person and their family carer and focusing on the individual's strengths, abilities and values (see Chapter 3). Even in the presence of chronic illness or multiple disabilities, nurses can use the strengths-based approach to respond to each individual's life changes and presenting clinical symptoms by focusing on their abilities and well-being. Health promotion outcomes can then be further enhanced based on people's strengths, abilities, aspirations, health and well-being.

The goal of health promotion for persons with altered health maintenance is to facilitate lifestyle changes by modifying thought patterns and behaviours and encouraging self-care in managing restoration and rehabilitation. More nursing research is required that shifts the emphasis from illness and disease to the expectation of wellness, even in the presence of chronic disease and functional impairment (Touhy & Jett, 2012). The strengths-based approach assumes that when clients are encouraged to use self-efficacy they become empowered to change their behaviour. When used with other models of health promotion, techniques that assist a strengths-based approach are more likely to achieve a positive health journey. These techniques are outlined in Table 5.1.

TABLE 5.1 *Techniques to assist a strengths-based approach in primary care*

STRENGTHS APPROACH AND TECHNIQUES TO ASSIST IMPLEMENTATION INTO PRACTICE	
Tenet	Techniques
Self-determination	Geriatric assessment that provides basis for individual patients to discuss the opportunities/skills they want to expand upon.
Empowerment	Health promotion techniques to encourage behaviour change and learning new skills.
Collaboration	Provide opportunities for clients to work together with other clients or/ and staff and families on a mutually agreed activity.
Reflection on change	Provide opportunity for staff to hear patients' stories and use opportunity to mutually identify areas for future development.
Community engagement	Encourage patients, staff and families to participate in community support programs targeted towards health promotion and healthy ageing.
Regeneration	Encourage sharing of success while providing support for ongoing opportunities through a shared time for discussion.

Using evidence-based nursing assessment tools

There is recognition in gerontological nursing that evidence-based assessment tools are essential to promote healthy ageing and improve the effectiveness of the delivery of health care. As described in Chapters 2, 3 and 4 a comprehensive geriatric assessment of an individual is defined broadly as a multidimensional process that incorporates an in-depth assessment of a person's physical, medical, psychological, cultural and social needs, capabilities and resources. The overall goal of assessment is to improve quality of life. Importantly nurses must have the skills to differentiate between normal changes of ageing and those caused by disease, the coexistence of multiple diseases and co-morbidities and under-reporting of symptoms by older people (Touhy & Jett, 2012). Evidence-based tools are further discussed in Chapters 8, 9 and 10.

The future of primary care in Australia and New Zealand

In Australia and New Zealand primary health care nurses already play an important role in medication management, including reviewing medication use in the context of a patient's health assessment or chronic disease plan, advising patients on quality use of medicines, helping to identify patients at risk of adverse events, contributing to the patient's health record, directly administering vaccines, and managing stores of medications and vaccines.

In future nurses in primary care practice will extend their skills in case management to coordinate multidisciplinary teams. Using the strengths-based approach gerontological nurses will optimise client self-care, improve continuity of care across settings, enhance clients' quality of life, decrease length of hospitalisation, increase client and staff satisfaction, and promote cost-effective use of scarce resources. Nurses will develop clinical decision making capacity beyond current models of evidence-based practice to include psychosocial, public health, marketing and ethics frameworks (Jutel, 2008).

Nurses in Australia and New Zealand can draw on research provided by bodies such as the US National Institute of Nursing Research (NINR), whose mission is to support the science that advances nursing knowledge. The main areas of research of the NINR currently are promoting health and preventing disease, improving quality of life, eliminating health disparities and setting directions for end of life research (Tabloski, 2010). The focus is on cost-effective, behavioural techniques, such as health promotion.

Nurses can develop evidence-based interventions identified as currently unavailable by the Cochrane Collection, such as decision making processes for older people facing the possibility of long-term care, the use of interactive health communication applications for people with chronic disease and promotion of a person-centred approach in clinical consultations (Cochrane Collaboration, 2014).

Professional development opportunities in primary care

The growing number of older people requires us to think differently about their potential care and support requirements and to work in co-partnership between health care providers and clients. Advanced nursing models such as the Nurse Practitioner Model will improve outcomes in primary care (Holm & Severinsson, 2013). Values-based nursing models of care such as strengths-based care offer the opportunity for older people, their families, carers and communities to identify and mobilise their strengths and resources so they can live a life that encourages empowerment and quality of life.

Gerontological nurses in practice have the opportunity to provide valuable primary care to older people by extending the traditional community nurse role to that of practice nurse, nurse practitioner and nurse manager (see Chapter 4). Advanced nursing knowledge will lead to improved leadership in implementing models of care focused on efficiency and effectiveness (Holm & Severinsson, 2013). As discussed in Chapter 4 implicit in these roles are the aspects of advocate, educator, manager, consultant and researcher. The gerontological nurse can also contribute to and participate in research by identifying clinical problems appropriate for study, gathering data and using research findings to develop evidence-based nursing interventions (Tabloski, 2010).

Increasingly nurse practice managers and NPs will work alongside community nurses, GPs and geriatricians in primary health to provide screening, holistic assessment and intervention strategies for older people, thus reducing duplication of services and providing continuity of care (Hunter, 2012). There is a growing demand for nurses who recognise the 'red flags' of the geriatric syndrome – such as mobility impairment, sensory impairment, cognitive impairment and incontinence – to implement strategies and use guidelines based on evidence-based, person-centred practice (Tolson, Booth & Schofield, 2011a; Touhy & Jett, 2012). In primary care rigorous assessment of functional health patterns becomes the basis for holistic assessment, representing the underlying physical, social, psychological and spiritual foundations of the individual and their relationship with the environment (Gordon, 1994). Nurses will also facilitate ethical non-coercive decision making by older adults, with family caregivers, for maintaining everyday living, receiving treatment, initiating advance directives and implementing end of life care (Touhy & Jett, 2012).

:ing the strengths-based approach in primary care

Case scenario 5.1

Since his wife died suddenly two years ago Mr Smith lives alone in a small cottage in a rural town. He has spent his life working hard as a machine operator in a local saw mill and, since retiring 10 years ago at the age of 70, has kept active in his garden as well as playing bowls. He has some signs of osteoarthritis, which is managed with regular Panadol. Mr Smith's general practitioner has requested the completion of Bill's annual health review by the community registered nurse.

You are a final year student nurse completing a three week placement in the community setting. You have visited Bill with the community registered nurse and you note a number of changes from Bill's previous functional assessment as follows:

› Bill's weight has decreased 10 kg in the past 12 months.

› Bill has mentioned that his bowel habits have changed in the past two months, with bouts of constipation followed by diarrhoea.

› When asked about sleep patterns Bill has explained that he wakes most nights and finds it difficult to get back to sleep as he has a pain in his back that 'gnaws at him'.

› When asked about exercise Bill mentions that he has given his bowls away as he is too tired in the afternoon and falls asleep in his chair. He has also been neglecting the garden as it is 'getting beyond him'.

❯ When asked how he is feeling about life generally Bill talks about his loneliness since his wife passed away and his lack of motivation to cook for himself or eat properly. Recently his close friend passed away and he is missing his company and social interaction.

❯ When asked about his family Bill explains that he does not want to bother his daughter, who lives 30 minutes away on a nearby farm and is 'busy with her own family'.

Reflective questions

Read and reflect on the case scenario of Bill and address the following questions:

❯ How would you approach Bill about his current situation?

❯ Using the strengths-based approach what techniques would you use to assist you in establishing Bill's capabilities?

❯ How would you develop a strategy with Bill to maintain his level of capability based on his wishes, values and preferences?

Reflective activity

Consider your nursing education and practice and think about the following:

● What other health professionals in the multidisciplinary team would you refer Bill to ensure he receives appropriate care tailored to his needs?

● Based on your interview with Bill what types of evidence-based screening tests would you consider as part of Bill's geriatric assessment?

Summary

● The development of primary care in Australia and New Zealand involves nurses providing health promotion, prevention and rehabilitative services.

● Evidence-based nursing interventions that promote health and wellness will be based on the best available current evidence to provide optimum outcomes for clients and their families.

● Innovative models of care will incorporate clinical decision making capacity with a strengths-based approach to care for older people.

● Gerontological nurses in primary practice will be expected to develop advanced practice and nurse practitioner skills and knowledge.

Conclusion

This chapter has outlined major developments for nurses in practice in the provision of primary clinical care for older people. In Australia and New Zealand aged care reform in the primary sector is still in its infancy. Nurses have the opportunity to make a significant contribution to the development of evidence-based models of care and interventions in primary care. The strengths-based approach to care provides the platform for nurses to achieve continuous improvement in providing the best outcomes for clients and families based on their values, preferences and experiences.

Further reading

You may like to take a look at the following reading recommendations:

- Australia's Department of Health: http://www.health.gov.au/
- Australian Institute of Health and Welfare: http://www.aihw.gov.au/

References

Australian Government Department of Health and Ageing. (2010). *Building a 21st Century Primary Health Care System: Australia's First National Primary Health Care Strategy*. Canberra.

Australian Health Ministers' Advisory Council. (2004). *Age-friendly Principles and Practices: Managing Older People in the Health Service Environment*. Melbourne: Victorian Government Department of Human Services.

Bodenheimer, T., Wagner, E. & Grumbach, J. (2002). Improving primary care for patients with chronic illness. *Journal of the American Medical Association*, 288(14), 1775–9.

Booth, J., Tolson, D., Schofield, I. & Lawrence, M. (2011). Applying the evidence to practice. In D. Tolson, J. Booth & I. Schofield (Eds.), *Evidence Informed Nursing with Older People*. Chichester: Wiley-Blackwell.

Chenoworth, L. (2010). Evidence-based nursing practice. In P. Brown (Ed.), *Health Care of the Older Adult: An Australian and New Zealand Nursing Perspective*. Warriewood, NSW: Woodslane Press Pty Ltd.

Cochrane Collaboration. (2014). Decision aids for people facing health treatment or screening decisions. doi: 10.1002/14651858.CD001431.pub4

Gillespie, L., Robertson, M., Gillespie, W., Lamb, W., Gates, S., Cumming, R. & Rowe, B. (2009). Interventions for preventing falls in older people living in the community. *Cochrane Database of Systematic Reviews*. doi: 10.1002/14651858.CD007146

Gordon, M. (1994). *Nursing Diagnosis: Process and Application*. St Louis: Mosby.

Holm, A. & Severinsson, E. (2013). Effective nursing leadership of older persons in the community – a systematic review. *Journal of Nursing Management*. doi: 10.1111/jonm.12076

Hunter, S. (2012). *Miller's Nursing for Wellness in Older Adults*. Philadelphia: Wolters Kluwer/Lippincott Williams & Wilkins.

Joanna Briggs Institute. (2011). *Joanna Briggs Institute Reviewer's Manual*. Adelaide.

Jutel, A. (2008). Beyond evidence-based nursing: Tools for practice. *Journal of Nursing Management*, 16, 417–421.

Kelly, I., Tolson, D., Schofield, I. & Booth, J. (2005). Describing gerontological nursing: An academic exercise or prerequisite for progress? *Journal of Clinical Nursing*. doi: 10.1111/j.1365–2702.2005.01147.x

King, A. (2001). *The Primary Health Care Strategy*. Retrieved from http://www.moh.govt.nz

Menec, V. & Nowicki, S. (2014). Examining the relationship between communities' 'age-friendliness' and life satisfaction and self-perceived health in rural Manitoba, Canada. *Rural and Remote Health*, 14, 2594.

New Zealand Guidance Group. (2003). *Assessment Processes for Older People*. Wellington.

Nursing and Midwifery Board of Australia. (2011). *Code of Ethics for Nurses*. Melbourne.

Pearson, A., Weeks, S. & Stern, C. (2010). *Translation Science and the JBI Model of Evidence-Based Healthcare*. Baltimore: Lippincott, Williams & Wilkins

Tabloski, P. (2010). *Gerontological Nursing*. (2nd edition). New Jersey: Pearson.

Tolson, D., Booth, J. & Schofield, I. (2011a). Principles of gerontological nursing. In D. Tolson, J. Booth & I. Schofield (Eds.), *Evidence Informed Nursing with Older People*. Oxford: Wiley-Blackwell.

Tolson, D., Booth, J. & Schofield, I. (2011b). *Evidence Informed Nursing with Older People*. Chichester: Wiley-Blackwell.

Touhy, T. & Jett, K. (2012). *Ebersole & Hess' Toward Healthy Ageing: Human Needs & Nursing Response*. St Louis: Elsevier.

World Health Organization. (2008). *Primary Health Care – Now More Than Ever. The World Health Report*. Geneva.

Part 2

Chronicity and ageing

6 Changing disease patterns

Wendy Moyle

Learning objectives

After reading this chapter you will be able to:

1 Define the key concepts of geriatric syndromes.

2 Discuss the impact of geriatric syndromes on ageing.

3 Discuss the relationship between population ageing and its effect on patterns of disease.

4 Define self-efficacy and the importance of self-efficacy for older people.

5 Define dementia and the influence of Alzheimer's disease and other dementias on ageing.

6 Define delirium and the relationship of delirium to ageing and dementia.

Introduction

This chapter looks at the complex and varied diseases of older age often referred to as the **geriatric syndrome** with a particular focus on diseases that impact on functional status; in particular **delirium**, falls and fractures, incontinence, and **Alzheimer's disease** and other **dementias**.

Population ageing is almost a worldwide phenomenon and certainly a common one in the western world. Population ageing refers to an increase in the proportion of older people (65 years and over) accompanied by a reduction in the proportion of children (15 years and younger), alongside a reduction in the proportion of people of working age. The most significant factor influencing population ageing is a reduction in the fertility rate, which is unlikely to rise to the high levels common in the past before adequate successful contraception. People are also living longer as a result of improved medical technology and nutrition, which helps to prevent or delay the onset of ageing changes. Population ageing has major consequences for society and in particular for health and care services.

Geriatric syndrome Occurs when the unique features of common health conditions in the elderly, such as delirium, falls, incontinence and frailty, are highly prevalent, multifactorial, and associated with substantial morbidity and poor outcomes.

Delirium An acute confused state lasting from hours to a few weeks.

Alzheimer's disease The most common type of dementia.

As discussed in Chapter 2 the proportion of older people has been steadily rising in the western world with increases in the proportion of older people and a decline in younger age groups. The proportion of people over 65 years of age in Australia in 2011 was just over 3.0 million, 13.5 per cent of the population (Australian Bureau of Statistics, 2013). New Zealand has also seen a boom in the 65 years and over population and at 635 200 this figure makes up 14 per cent of the New Zealand population (Statistics New Zealand, 2013). Although ageing is not necessarily synonymous with illness, infirmity or frailty, it does correlate with disability, impairment and handicap (Heitkemper, 2005). Chapter 2 demonstrates this further with an outline of ageing as a risk factor for disability and chronic disease as well as the implications of the rising number of those over 85 years, reported as the old-old population.

> **Dementia**
> An umbrella term used to describe a collection of symptoms caused by disorders affecting the brain.
>
> **Population ageing** Refers to an increase in the proportion of older people accompanied by a reduction in the proportion of children, alongside a reduction in the proportion of people of working age.

Ageing and frailty

The concepts of ageing and ageing theories are discussed in Chapter 1. In this chapter ageing will be examined in the context of **frailty**. Ageing was defined by Fedarko (2011, p. 27) as 'the decline and deterioration of functional properties at the cellular, tissue and organ level'. This decline increases older people's vulnerability to disease and mortality. It also increases functional decline due to injury, disease and falls. Frailty is defined as 'a state of vulnerability to poor resolution of homeostasis after a stressor event and it is a consequence of cumulative decline in many physiological systems' (Clegg et al., 2013, p. 752). Approximately one in five older people (19%) in the 2011 Australian census had a need for assistance with one of the core everyday activities of daily living (Australian Bureau of Statistics, 2013). This rate was higher for women (22%) than for men (16%), and in both genders the need for assistance increased as they aged. The frailty rate of older people in New Zealand has been estimated to be lower at approximately 8.1 per cent (Barrett et al., 2006). In all cases the degree of severe or profound activity restriction is positively correlated with frailty. One fifth of older people aged 65 and over in Australia have a severe or profound activity restriction and it is predicted that the number in this group will rise by almost 100 per cent over the next two decades (Australian Institute of Health and Welfare, 2007).

> **Frailty** 'A state of vulnerability to poor resolution of homeostasis after a stressor event and it is a consequence of cumulative decline in many physiological systems' (Clegg et al., 2013, p. 752).

Although there is no clear-cut age where people become frail, acute and chronic illness can push the older person, and in particular the old-old, into a frail state. As discussed in Chapters 1 and 2 older people can also become frail without having a chronic disease state, and there is great variation in the onset of the ageing process and its rate and extent of progression. In this context frailty is an important and common geriatric syndrome.

Successful ageing

Frailty has often been used as a synonym for the increasing infirmities that accompany chronological ageing. However, this focus fails to consider that older individuals make personal meaning of their own frailty. It also ignores the fact that successful ageing requires a positive view of this unique stage of life. People who age successfully are thought to be those who adapt to the increasing biological and environmental restrictions of ageing (Baltes & Baltes, 1990). Similarly a nursing focus on the strengths and abilities of the older person encourages the older person to remain involved in the decision making process related to their care. Chapter 3 discusses the strengths-based approach and its implications for care of older people.

Geriatric syndrome

A **syndrome** is a group of signs and symptoms that occur together and characterise a particular condition. The underlying cause of the syndrome might not be known even when symptoms are present. The term 'geriatric syndrome' has been coined to highlight the unique features of common health conditions in older people that do not fit into discrete disease categories (Inouye et al., 2007). The most common geriatric syndromes are delirium, falls, incontinence and, as already mentioned, frailty. These conditions are highly prevalent in older people, especially in the frail older person and the old-old. There are multiple underlying factors that contribute to the geriatric syndrome and these may involve multiple organ systems. Previous research suggests that some geriatric syndromes might share a common group of risk factors and these may lead to frailty (Tinetti et al., 2005). Frailty is characterised as a state of decreased physiological reserve and increased vulnerability (Fried et al., 2001). In geriatric assessment an older person is considered to be frail when they have three or more of the following: unintentional weight loss, weakness defined by grip

> **Syndrome**
> A group of signs and symptoms that occur together and characterise a particular condition.

strength, low physical activity and slowed motor performance (Fried et al., 2001).

As a result of frailty the older person is more at risk of adverse health outcomes that can result in hospitalisation, frequently as a result of falls and disability, and nursing home placement and mortality (Bandeen-Roche et al., 2006). Therefore, as already acknowledged in Chapter 2, the human, economic and societal impact from this syndrome is enormous. Rehabilitation programs have been considered to be the best option for maintaining and restoring functional ability in older people following a fall or disability, even for the 'old-old'. There are other factors that also influence rehabilitation. Personal **self-efficacy**, expressed as the ability of the person to regulate their motivation, thought processes and emotional states through appropriate behavioural changes, can affect the older person's functional status during rehabilitation (Tung, Cooke & Moyle, 2013). Positive self-identity in late life can also assist the older person to see themselves as adaptive rather than disabled (Gilleard & Higgs, 2000) and this will also encourage active rehabilitation. Using a strengths-based nursing approach the nurse will support the older person to maintain optional independence by encouraging the older person to work with their strengths. As indicated earlier the most common geriatric syndromes are delirium, falls and incontinence. The next section of this chapter will discuss each of these syndromes.

Self-efficacy
The ability of the person to regulate their motivation, thought processes and emotional states, and appropriate behavioural changes. Self-efficacy affects the older person's functional status during rehabilitation.

Delirium

Delirium is a clinical syndrome associated with an acute decline in cognitive function. Delirium is an acute confused state lasting from hours to a few weeks. It is characterised by changes in the sleep–wake cycle, attention, perception, thinking, memory and psychomotor behaviour (Meako, Thompson & Cochrane, 2011). Delirium also frequently occurs following major surgery, such as orthopaedic surgery (Meako, Thompson & Cochrane, 2011). Although a common syndrome, it is often overlooked and misdiagnosed as dementia, psychosis or depression. One of the factors influencing whether a patient receives an assessment for delirium is the fact that nurses are not adept at assessing and recognising changes in a patient's cognitive status (Moyle et al., 2011a). Delirium can occur in older people across settings, in particular in acute and long-term care.

Delirium is usually seen on day one or day two post-surgery and can result in increased morbidity and prolonged stay in the acute setting (Sykes, 2012).

Furthermore, people who experience delirium can be subjected to an increased use of chemical and physical restraints and increased losses in functional ability (Meako, Thompson & Cochrane, 2011). In acute care settings a mix of both surgical and intrinsic risk factors are involved in the development of delirium. The most common predisposing risk factors include advanced age, vision and/or hearing deficits, impaired cognitive function (people with dementia are at increased risk of developing delirium and this is called delirium superimposed on dementia (DSD)), and co-morbid medical and/or psychiatric disease states including depression (Fick et al., 2009). Precipitating factors include fluid and electrolyte imbalance, infection, poor pain control and medications (Fick et al., 2009). Facilitating factors can include environmental, social and lifestyle situations that influence the patient's comfort (Fick et al., 2009). Environmental factors might be noise and light, while social and lifestyle factors can include involvement of friends and family (see Table 6.1).

TABLE 6.1 *Summary of risk factors for delirium*

PATIENT CHARACTERISTICS	PATHOLOGY	ENVIRONMENT	ACUTE ILLNESS
Age	Cognitive impairment	No visible daylight	Temperature
Visual impairment	Chronic depression	No clock	Infection
Hearing deficits	Cardiac disease	No visitors	Sedation
History of alcohol abuse	Pulmonary disease	Isolation	Dehydration
Sleep disturbances	Diabetes	Physical restraint	Electrolyte imbalance
History of falls			Duration of anaesthesia
			Duration of surgery

Prevention and management of delirium includes preoperative assessment of the patient's status, early diagnosis, and interventions to right the cause of the delirium; that is, antibiotics for infection and non-pharmacological interventions such as involvement of family and friends to help the person regain cognitive awareness. The best instrument for assessing for a state of delirium is the Confusion Assessment Method (CAM) (Inouye et al., 1990). Assessment includes identification of recent changes in the person's thinking and memory. Ongoing assessment is necessary while an alteration in cognitive function persists.

While the recent focus in the nursing literature has been on the identification of delirium in the acute care setting, it is important for nurses to recognise that delirium may also arise in older people in long-term care settings. Delirium in the long-term care setting is often related to an infection, such as a urinary tract or respiratory infection. The nurse working in long-term care must continue to monitor and assess the older person for signs of delirium and outcomes of treatment.

Falls and fractures

Falls, and as a consequence of them, fractures, are associated with frailty and impaired limb and movement function. Falls are common with around one third of those 65 years and over falling at least once yearly (Moylan & Binder, 2007). The estimated number of hospitalised cases in Australia due to falls in people 65 and over in 2009–2010 was 83 800 (Bradley, 2013). The numbers are similar in New Zealand with between 22 and 60 per cent of people over 65 years sustaining a fall each year (Accident Compensation Corporation, 2012). Falls are more common in women: 69 per cent of cases in 2009–10 (Bradley, 2013). This number has continued to rise alongside the increase in the proportion of the older population. Falls also increase with age, with the highest rate of falls being in those aged 95 years and older (Bradley, 2013).

The most common fracture as a result of a fall is a fracture of the neck of the femur. Osteoporosis is characterised by low bone mass and is common in more than 60 per cent of people over 70 years of age and may contribute to a bone fracture (Rosenzweig & Mishra, 2009). A fracture associated with osteoporosis is known as a 'fragility fracture' (Rosenzweig & Mishra, 2009). Older people can also develop anxiety following a fall, even if they don't develop a fracture, and as a result this may reduce their activities and can interfere with their quality of life.

A strengths-based approach to falls

Using a strengths-based approach nurses can help the patient overcome falls anxiety by encouraging a focus away from the problem of fear of falling by seeking an understanding of the person and their family's strengths, and helping them to build on those strengths. The nurse can also assist by helping the patient's understanding of the science behind a fear of falling so that they can mobilise their resources to overcome their fear. The nurse in this situation will provide support, teach the patient and family ways to overcome the fear of falling, and guide and encourage the patient's progress. Where the patient feels they are being treated as a partner in their care rather than a patient that the nurse needs to manage, they are more likely to be involved and want to develop or strengthen their competencies.

Prevention of falls

There is ongoing evidence suggesting that, while falls are common as we age, many can be prevented. Human balance is influenced by the interaction of multiple sensory, motor and integrative systems (Lord, Smith & Menant, 2010). As we age these systems are thought to decline and as a result can influence falls in older people. Exercises that reduce the chance of falling include challenging and progressive weight-bearing balance exercises (Lord, Smith & Menant, 2010).

elirium following a fall

Case scenario 6.1

Martha is 87 years of age. She was admitted to the acute hospital following a fall at home that required surgery for a fractured femur. Martha appeared to be doing well post-surgery but on day two Martha appeared sleepier than usual, and she was disorientated in time and place, and mistook one of the staff for her daughter. Martha was not paying attention when staff communicated with her. She spent her time staring into space and reaching out into the air, as if she saw something to reach out to.

Martha's family were called in and they reported that Martha had no history of memory problems, or depression. A CAM assessment suggested Martha had delirium, possibly as a result of the duration of anaesthesia and surgery and her post-surgical pain. A further physical assessment was conducted and a decision was made to increase Martha's analgesia, to continue with

regular CAM assessment, and to have a family member sit and talk with Martha, to show her photographs of her family and house as a means to help her overcome her confusion. Martha's condition settled with no further complications and she was discharged to rehabilitation before returning to live with her daughter.

Reflective questions

Read and reflect on this case scenario and address the following questions:

> Could Martha's delirium have been prevented?

> What could the nursing staff have done to prepare Martha's family for her delirium?

> What environmental factors may have contributed to the development of Martha's delirium?

> Using a strengths-based approach how could staff approach the care of Martha?

Urinary incontinence

Urinary incontinence (UI) is defined as an inability to control the flow of urine that results in involuntary urination. The prevalence of UI is around 30 per cent in older people who live in the community and it rises to 50 per cent among older people who live in long-term care settings (Dey, 1997; Hellstrom et al., 1990). UI may occur

Urinary incontinence
An inability to control the flow of urine that results in involuntary urination.

independently or may be associated with dementia, a stroke or type 2 diabetes (Strandberg et al., 2013). This condition influences the well-being and autonomy of older people and in particular it influences the person who has a mobility deficit. To help reduce an older person's anxiety about urinary incontinence the nurse can help with education about the stimulants that may be causing the incontinence, information about bladder emptying and an awareness of where toilets are situated when the person is not in familiar surroundings.

There are three types of urinary incontinence. **Stress incontinence** is the loss of urine when pressure is exerted on the bladder by coughing, sneezing, laughing, exercising or lifting something heavy. Stress incontinence occurs when the sphincter muscle of the bladder has been weakened as a result of pregnancy or menopause, or the removal of the prostate gland in men. **Urge incontinence** is a sudden, intense urge to urinate, followed by an involuntary loss of urine. Urge incontinence may be caused by infection, bladder irritants such as coffee, or neurological conditions such as Parkinson's disease. **Overflow incontinence** is a result of an inability to fully empty the bladder, resulting in frequent small volumes of urine being released. **Mixed incontinence** is a mixture of different types of incontinence. **Functional incontinence** occurs as a result of impairment stopping the person getting to the toilet on time. Finally, **total incontinence** is uncontrollable leaking of urine.

> **Stress incontinence**
> The loss of urine when pressure is exerted on the bladder.
>
> **Urge incontinence**
> Sudden, intense urge to urinate, followed by an involuntary loss of urine.
>
> **Overflow incontinence**
> Result of an inability to fully empty the bladder, resulting in frequent small volumes of urine being released.
>
> **Mixed incontinence**
> A mixture of different types of incontinence.
>
> **Functional incontinence**
> Occurs as a result of impairment stopping the person getting to the toilet on time.
>
> **Total incontinence**
> Uncontrollable leaking of urine.

Independence and autonomy

The disorders outlined have helped to raise societal concern about the effects an ageing population will have on care services as well as whether there will be adequate numbers of trained staff to care for them. In particular the geriatric syndrome has raised fears about the potential cost of services for older people. There is research, however, that suggests this fear is unfounded. Nicholson (2009, p. 11) argues that 'the predominant models of frailty, rooted in physical deficit, decontextualize the meanings and over-simplify the experience' portrayed by frail, older people. As discussed in Chapter 2 in spite of society fears about frailty and ageing, research has shown that older people are realistic about their health and expectations and such expectations can positively affect the ageing process (Sarkisian et al., 2006). Older people use a number of strategies including maintaining community connections and relationships, and keeping active. They achieve resilience through a focus on emotional, practical and spiritual coping to get them through challenging situations that include progressive frailty and the syndromes described in this chapter (Moyle et al., 2010). The independence and autonomy of older people are the key links to the provision of nursing care that should focus on patients' capabilities and strengths so that nursing care concerns 'doing with' rather than 'doing for' them.

Resilience alongside frailty

Case scenario 6.2

Joan is 87 and lives on her own in Sydney. Joan was married for 60 years until her husband died seven years ago. Her husband's family remains in contact by telephone but daily support is from friends and neighbours. Joan had one son, Keith, who died of cancer while in his forties. Joan required major heart surgery five years ago. She recovered well but requires medication and visits her GP and attends outpatients regularly. In 2007 she fell and broke her ankle. The ankle joint did not mend well and she remained immobile for six months. During this time she was cared for at home by home and community care services twice a day and by a network of friends. Although she got back on her feet, Joan fell again, breaking her wrist on the second occasion. This left her unconfident, using a walking stick and unwilling to go out on her own. Very soon, however, in spite of pain, Joan was keen to go out into her garden and to meet socially with friends. This was the driver for Joan and she soon was going over the road to visit her neighbour, aged 91. Thus, Joan continued to prosper and her mobility improved to the point where she required fewer support services.

Reflective questions

Read and reflect on this case scenario and address the following questions:

> Have you experienced older people such as Joan? If so, what has driven them to keep on going even in the event of adversity, such as chronic illness?

> If you were the home and community care registered nurse how might you approach the care of Joan using a strengths-based approach?

(Case scenario adapted and published with permission of Caroline Nicholson, 2009, p. 281.)

One of the diseases affecting older people is Alzheimer's disease (AD) and other types of dementia. The following section explores AD and the common dementias.

Alzheimer's disease and other dementias

'Dementia' is an umbrella term used to describe a collection of symptoms caused by disorders affecting the brain and often described as a syndrome.

There is no one specific disease that causes this disorder and it is not a clinical diagnosis itself without an underlying disease or disorder, for example AD. Dementia affects thinking, behaviour and the ability to perform everyday tasks of daily living. Although dementia increases with age, it is not a normal part of ageing. As we age we may notice poorer short-term memory as we slowly lose brain cells. This is normal and is referred to as age-related decline, not dementia.

In 2010, globally there were approximately 35.6 million people living with dementia, with a further 7.7 million new cases predicted annually (World Health Organization, 2012). Access Economics has projected a four-fold increase in the number of cases of dementia in Australia from 2009 to 2050, an increase from 245 000 to 1.1 million people (Access Economics, 2011). New Zealand will see a similar pattern of increase, but in Asia, where the population is rapidly ageing, there will be even more dramatic increases in the number of cases of dementia (Draper, 2011). As a result of these projections Access Economics (2009) also projected that dementia will become the third greatest source of health and aged care expenditure within the next two decades, and by 2060 they predict that dementia will far exceed expenditure on any other health condition. In Australia, these predictions led to the development in 2005 of what is termed the 'Dementia Initiative', which made dementia a national health priority and established three dementia collaborative research centres to support research and service development. Dementia training and study centres were also established to train health care professionals and 'Dementia Essentials' was established to train care workers. Furthermore, the Dementia Behaviour Management Advisory Service (DBMAS) is an Australian government initiative and was established for support and advice on best practice in behaviour management (see http://dbmas.org.au). The DBMAS service is offered in all states and territories of Australia and is accessible to staff, family and also care providers. The DBMAS service aims to improve the quality of life of people with dementia and their carers.

Young onset dementia This refers to people with onset of dementia before 65 years of age.

Dementia is more common in people who are 65 years and older. However, it can also happen to people in their 40s and 50s and this is referred to as **young onset dementia**. Neurodegenerative disease, which is defined as progressive brain cell death, is the cause of most dementias. Dementia is a progressive disorder that has three stages, although there is overlap between stages and it can be difficult to define these. The first stage is mild cognitive impairment. In this stage there is evidence of cognitive deterioration over time, although the individual is able to maintain basic activities of daily living. Depression and apathy can occur in this stage and can be accompanied by mood swings. The next stage is moderate impairment. In this stage there is persistent memory loss, forgetfulness about personal history and an inability to recognise family and friends. The person may become lost in familiar surroundings, experience mood and sleep disturbances, mobility and coordination is a challenge, and they can exhibit behavioural symptoms. The final stage is severe dementia. The person has lost the ability to recall, communicate or process information. Verbal communication is challenged and mobility is further challenged with the potential for falls. The person exhibits extreme problems with mood and behaviour and they are incontinent and have swallowing difficulties. As discussed in Chapter 2 the number of cases of dementia will continue to rise alongside the ageing of the population.

The most common type of dementia is AD, accounting for approximately 60 to 70 per cent of all cases (World Health Organization, 2012). AD can also occur in combination with any of the other forms of dementia. Vascular dementia is the second most common type of dementia, accounting for 15 to 20 per cent of cases, followed by frontotemporal dementia, which occurs in 5 to 10 per cent of cases, and dementia with Lewy bodies, which occurs in up to 5 per cent of cases (Draper, 2011). Conditions that can cause dementia include Parkinson's disease, Huntington's disease and Korsakoff's syndrome, which is alcohol related dementia (see Table 6.2).

Early signs of dementia

Early signs of dementia include a progressive decline in memory and thinking that results in significant impairment of daily living function. Dementia affects other brain functions and results in the person suffering from disorientation, impaired comprehension, a reduction in learning capacity, difficulties with calculating ability, language, judgement, reasoning and information processing. Families often comment that prior to diagnosis they notice the individual having difficulty with word finding, confusion particularly when the individual is in an unfamiliar setting, and personality changes such as being aggressive, displaying apathy or withdrawing from favourite activities. While memory loss and word finding are of most concern in the early stages, as the dementia progresses other symptoms develop and become more troublesome, such as wandering and functional urinary incontinence (see Table 6.3).

TABLE 6.2 *Types of dementia*

TYPES OF DEMENTIA	CHARACTERISTICS	SYMPTOMS	BRAIN CHANGES
Alzheimer's disease	Most common type of dementia. Accounts for 60–70% of all cases of dementia. Progressive degenerative illness. Almost all people with Down syndrome will develop AD.	Early symptoms: difficulty remembering names and recent events; apathy and depression. Later symptoms: impaired judgement; disorientation; confusion; behaviour changes; difficulties with speech, swallowing and walking.	Deposits of beta-amyloid (plaques) and tau (tangles) as well as evidence of nerve cell damage and death in the brain.
Vascular dementia	Second most common type of dementia. Individuals can have mixed dementia – two or more types of dementia.	Early symptoms: impaired judgement; inability to plan to complete a task	Brain injury as a result of bleeding and blood vessel blockage.
Dementia with Lewy bodies (DLB)		Early symptoms: sleep disturbance; visual hallucinations; muscle rigidity; large fluctuations in attention and thinking.	Abnormal clumps of the protein alpha-synuclein
Parkinson's disease		Early symptoms: problems with movement; if dementia develops, symptoms are similar to DLB.	Abnormal clumps of the protein alpha-synuclein in the substantia nigra. Thought to cause degeneration of the nerve cells that produce dopamine.
Frontotemporal dementia (Pick's disease)	Usually develops at a younger age, around 60.	Changes in personality and behaviour; language difficulties; difficulty recognising objects, understanding or expressing language.	Involves degeneration in one or both of the frontal or temporal lobes of the brain.
Wernicke-Korsakoff syndrome	Chronic memory disorder caused by severe deficiency of thiamine (vitamin B-1). Usually caused by alcohol abuse and usually irreversible.	Memory problems; personality changes; visual and auditory hallucinations; lack of insight.	When thiamine levels fall too low, brain cells do not function.

TABLE 6.3 *Common presenting complaints in dementia*

Losses	Memory impairment
	Word finding difficulty
	Decline in self-care
	Decline in management of financial affairs
	Decline in work and activity performance
Changes in behaviour	Withdrawal and isolation
	Personality change
	Mood change, e.g. often depressed mood
	Behaviour that is not usual for the individual
	Paranoid ideas, e.g. someone is stealing money

Dementia care

The care and financial cost of people with dementia puts enormous strain on families, society and care services. Behavioural and psychological symptoms of dementia (BPSD) are common and in particular in mid to late stages of dementia. Symptoms of BPSD, such as aggression and agitation, can increase the challenge of care provision and can reduce relationships the person may have had with family and/or care staff.

Society, health professionals and governments recognise AD and other dementias as a major public health concern. Although most dementias are irreversible there has been advancement in drug treatments offering temporary assistance in slowing down the progress of the disease. These treatments are cholinesterase inhibitor drugs such as donepezil (Aricept) and rivastigmine (Exelon). Although there are a number of international clinical trials of new treatments there is currently no cure for AD or other dementias and there is nothing known to provide a cure in the immediate future. The interest in psychosocial treatments has therefore increased as a means of helping to overcome some of the BPSDs and improve quality of life.

The majority of people with dementia live in the community in their own home. Family carers offer an important contribution, in particular emotional support, in the early stages of the disease followed by physical support as the disease progresses. The number of community services available for support has grown over the last decade and such services assist both the person with dementia and the family carer to allow the person to stay at home as long as possible. Carers of people with dementia commonly delay accessing formal community support until a crisis occurs (Witucki Brown et al., 2007). Nurses play a pivotal role in encouraging families and people with dementia to work together and, alongside community support staff, will help to play an important role in managing their quality of life and care (Mittelman, 2008). The role of the family carer is further discussed in Chapter 8.

Dementia and strengths-based care

As the disease progresses and the demands for physical care become greater there is often little choice but to place the person with dementia into long-term aged care. There are various types of care within such settings and, depending on availability and the physical needs of the person, they will be placed into a low or high care setting or, if they exhibit BPSD that may disturb other residents, or they are at risk of harm from wandering, they may be placed into a special care unit that focuses on care of people with dementia. Chapter 4 discusses the different types of care available for care of older people.

Dementia can undermine the person with dementia's self-esteem and feelings of self-worth (Preston, Marshall & Bucks, 2007). However, when society values the person with dementia and positions them as individuals of worth, this will contribute towards improving their quality of life (Jennings 2004; Moyle et al., 2014; Moyle et al., 2011b; Sabat, 2001). It is imperative that the family carer and the work that they do in caring for the person with dementia is also valued (Moyle et al., 2014).

Despite the belief that people with dementia have limited quality of life recent research suggests that factors influencing a positive quality of life are related to positive relationships with family, staff and others; with some control over aspects of life and feeling they are contributing to society (Moyle et al., 2011b). A strengths-based approach will focus on positive relationships and help the family caregiver build such a relationship with care staff. This may help to overcome some of the tensions that can arise when the person with dementia enters long-term care (Moyle, Edwards & Clinton, 2002). The literature also indicates that the way family caregivers see their role once the person with dementia is placed in a nursing home and the way staff also approach the family caregiver will influence the way they contribute to the care of their family member (Bramble et al., 2009). Care staff can also contribute to a person's quality of life by focusing on the strengths and capabilities of the person (Moyle et al., 2013). An individual's strengths and capabilities can be strengthened through the way we perceive and approach a person with dementia.

There are many different personae that individuals have, whether they have a diagnosis of dementia or not. They can be a mother, father, neighbour, friend, teacher, to name but a few. Each of these personae demand different distinct types of behaviour, but to achieve these types of behaviour the individual must be seen through one of these personae rather than as an individual with no hope because they have a diagnosis of dementia (Sabat, 2001). Positioning of the person with dementia can, within a social situation and conversation, place the individual as a patient needing help ('Hello, this is George. He has Alzheimer's disease'), or can position an individual as someone who can have some control over their life ('Hello George, what would you like to do now?'). In particular in our professional lives we see what we expect to see; an individual with a diagnosis and therefore unable to take control and requiring help. We also interpret the meaning of our experience in light of our prior expectations and therefore it is important that we demonstrate care that treats individuals with respect and dignity and positions the individual as the person they are, rather than as a disease process (Sabat, 2001).

The dementia diagnosis

A lack of understanding of the consequences of a diagnosis of dementia is not uncommon. Limited understanding of dementia, its long-term effects and sources of support can make management and coping with dementia difficult. A diagnosis of dementia affects both the person with the diagnosis and family and friends in their network. Coping with dementia necessitates fundamental changes in one's life as well as one's supports. While people with dementia have individual reactions to a diagnosis, there are some who experience low self-esteem and feel disempowered (Burgener & Berger, 2008); while for others once over the initial shock of the diagnosis they are capable of adjusting to the diagnosis. Case scenario 6.3 of Kim demonstrates her resilience and coping with a dementia diagnosis. Maintaining a sense of identity, being consulted and actively participating in decision making are key components influencing coping for people with dementia (Preston, Marshall & Bucks, 2007). A strengths-based care approach will focus on these characteristics as a way of encouraging and mentoring the person/family to manage their situation.

A focus on the good things in life

Case scenario 6.3

Kim was diagnosed five years ago at the age of 53 with younger onset frontal temporal dementia. At the time of diagnosis she reacted with sadness and cried day and night for a month. Although her life has been far from smooth since diagnosis, she has used her situation to strengthen her resilience and to drive herself forward to achieve more of her goals and to live each day as though it is her last, just in case it is. She does not want to be defined by the symptoms of her disease – but rather as a wife, mother and friend. Rather than waiting for the inevitable, Kim has continued to study and completed a degree in psychology, something that had long been on her bucket list. She plans every detail of her day and uses reminders in all parts of her daily life – on her computer, telephone and calendar – to keep her life controllable and to assist with her memory loss. She believes in informing others about dementia and reminding others of the reasons why dementia is an important health priority. She writes a daily blog about her experience to help society understand the condition, as a reminder that she is a person with personal interests, and that she is not just a disease. She keeps active through engagement with an Alzheimer's Association and regular meetings and discussions with friends and family. Her focus on the good things in life, spending quality time with her family, pursuing more of her goals and dreams, and looking beyond herself have allowed her to see her life as interesting, busy and fulfilling even in the adversity of a dementia diagnosis.

Reflective questions

Read and reflect on this case scenario and address the following questions:

> Have you experienced people such as Kim in your practice or readings?

> What has helped Kim to take such a positive approach to life?

> What can we do to help others in similar situations to strengthen their resilience?

Reflective activity

Consider your nursing education and practice and reflect on the following:

- Do you see examples of geriatric syndrome in your practice and/or education? If so what are the examples you have seen? How have these situations/people been managed in practice? How might a strengths-based care approach improve opportunities for people such as Kim?
- Can you think of examples where there have been good examples of assessment and management of geriatric syndrome and/or people with dementia? What were the characteristics of these good examples? How might we ensure such characteristics are common practice in health care settings?
- Have you seen examples of people with delirium? What made you realise the person had delirium rather than dementia or depression for example? What type of assessment was used to detect delirium?

Summary

- The most common syndromes that are referred to as being part of the geriatric syndrome are delirium, falls and incontinence.

- Older people have an individual response to ageing.

- Population ageing has had an impact on the number of older people and as a result an increase in chronic disease and disability such as incontinence.

- Older people respond differently to having a disability; however, positive self-efficacy and image will encourage the individual to respond positively to ageing.

- The number of cases of Alzheimer's disease and other dementias has increased alongside an ageing population.

- The increase in Alzheimer's disease and other dementias will impact on the burden of care.

Conclusion

This chapter has examined population ageing and the influence of ageing on frailty. Furthermore, an exploration of the geriatric syndrome and the common syndromes associated with the geriatric syndrome are outlined. The chapter finishes with an overview of Alzheimer's disease and the other dementias and recommends that health professionals concentrate on individual strengths and capabilities as well as provision of care that is respectful and considers the individual's dignity.

Further reading

You may also like to refer to the following reading that explores further the diversity among older Australians. This document focuses on the change over time of older people in Australian capital cities: Australian Institute of Health and Welfare. (2004). *Diversity among older Australians in capital cities 1996–2011*. Canberra. Retrieved from http://www.aihw.gov.au/publication-detail/?id=6442467629

References

Access Economics. (2009). *Keeping Dementia Front of Mind: Incidence and Prevalence 2009–2050*. Access Economics/Alzheimer's Australia.

Access Economics. (2011). *Dementia Across Australia: 2011–2050*. Access Economics/Alzheimer's Australia.

Accident Compensation Corporation (ACC). (2012). *Falls. Information for Health Professionals*. Retrieved from http://www.acc.co.nz/preventing-injuries/at-home/older-people/information-for-health-professionals/index.htm

Australian Bureau of Statistics. (2013). *Reflecting a Nation: Stories from the 2011 Census, 2012–2013*. Canberra.

Australian Institute of Health and Welfare. (2007). *Older Australia at a Glance* (4th edition). Canberra.

Baltes, P. & Baltes, M. (1990). *Successful Aging: Perspectives from the Behavioural Sciences*. Cambridge: Cambridge University Press.

Bandeen-Roche, K., Xue, Q., Ferrucci, L., Walston, J., Guralnik, J., Chaves, P., … Fried, L. (2006). Phenotype of frailty: Characterization in the women's health and aging studies. *Journals of Gerontology A Series*, 61(3), 262–6.

Barrett, P., Twitchin, S., Kletchko, S. & Faye, R. (2006). The living environments of community-dwelling older people who become frail: Another look at the Living Standards of Older New Zealanders Survey. *Social Policy Journal of New Zealand*, 28, 133–57.

Bradley, C. (2013). *Hospitalisations Due to Falls by Older People, Australia 2009–10. Injury Research and Statistics Series No. 70*. Canberra: AIHW.

Bramble, M., Moyle, W. & McAllister, M. (2009). Seeking connection: Family care experiences following long term dementia care placement. *Journal of Clinical Nursing*, 18, 3118–25.

Burgener, S. & Berger, B. (2008). Measuring perceived stigma in persons with progressive neurological disease. *Dementia: The International Journal of Social Research and Practice*, 7(1), 31–53.

Clegg, A., Young, J., Illiffe, S., Olde, M. & Rockwood, K. (2013). Frailty in elderly people. *The Lan.*, 381, 752–62.

Dey, A. (1997). Characteristics of elderly nursing home residents: Data from the 1995 National Nursing Home Survey. *Advance Data*, 2, 1–8.

Draper, B. (2011). *Understanding Alzheimer's and Other Dementias*. Woollahra, NSW: Longueville Books.

Fedarko, N. (2011). The biology of aging and frailty. *Clinical Geriatric Medicine*, 27, 27–37.

Fick, D., Kloanowski, A., Beattie, E. & McCrow, J. (2009). Delirium in early-stage Alzheimer's disease. Enhancing cognitive reserve as a possible preventive measure. *Journal of Gerontological Nursing*, 35(3), 1–14.

Fried, P., Tangen, C., Walston, J., Newman, A., Hirsch, C., Gottdiener, J., ... McBurnie, M. (2001). Frailty in older adults: Evidence for a phenotype. *Journals of Gerontology Series A*, 56A(3), M1–M11.

Gilleard, C. & Higgs, P. (2000). *Cultures of Ageing: Self, Citizen and the Body*. Harlow: Prentice Hall.

Heitkemper, M. (2005). *Older Adults*. Marrickville: Elsevier.

Hellstrom, L., Ekelund, P., Milsom, I. & Mellstrom, D. (1990). The prevalence of urinary incontinence and use of incontinence aids in 85-year-old men and women. *Age Ageing*, 19, 383–9.

Inouye, S., Studenski, S., Tinetti, M. & Kuchel, G. (2007). Geriatric syndromes: Clinical, research and policy implications of a core geriatric concept. *Journal of the American Geriatrics Society*, 55, 780–91.

Inouye, S., van Dyck, C., Alessi, C., Balkin, S., Siegal, A. & Horwitz, R. (1990). Clarifying confusion: The confusion assessment method. A new method for detection of delirium. *Annals of Internal Medicine*, 113(12), 941–8.

Jennings, B. (2004). Alzheimer's disease and the quality of life. In K. Doka (Ed.), *Living with Grief: Alzheimer's Disease*. Washington, DC: Hospice Foundation of America.

Lord, S., Smith, S. & Menant, J. (2010). Vision and falls in older people: Risk factors and intervention strategies. *Clinical Geriatric Medicine*, 26(4), 569–81.

Meako, M., Thompson, H. & Cochrane, B. (2011). Orthopaedic nurses' knowledge of delirium in older hospitalized patients. *Orthopaedic Nursing*, 30(4), 241–8.

Mittelman, M. (2008). Psychosocial intervention research: Challenges, strategies and measurement issues. *Aging & Mental Health*, 12, 1–14.

Moylan, K. & Binder, E. (2007). Falls in older adults: Risk assessment, management and prevention. *American Journal of Medicine*, 120, 493–7.

Moyle, W., Borbasi, S., Wallis, M., Olorenshaw, R. & Gracia, N. (2011a). Acute care management of older people with dementia: A qualitative perspective. *Journal of Clinical Nursing*, 20, 420–8.

Moyle, W., Clarke, C., Gracia, N., Reed, J., Cook, G,. Klein, B., ... Richardson, E. (2010). Older people maintaining mental health wellbeing through resilience: An appreciative inquiry study in four countries. *Journal of Nursing and Healthcare of Chronic Illness*, 2, 113–21.

Moyle, W., Edwards, H. & Clinton, M. (2002). Living with loss: Dementia and the family caregiver. *Australian Journal of Advanced Nursing*, 19(3), 25–31.

Moyle, W., Murfield, J., Venturato, L., Griffiths, S., Grimbeek, P., McAllister, M. & Marshall, J. (2014) Dementia and its influence on quality of life and what it means to be valued: Family members perceptions. *Dementia: The International Journal of Social Research and Practice*, 13(3), 412–25.

Moyle, W., Venturato, L., Cooke, M., Hughes, J., van Wyk, S. & Marshall, J. (2013). Promoting value in dementia care: Staff, resident and family experience of the capability model of dementia care. *Aging and Mental Health*. doi:10.1080/1360786 3.2012.758233

Moyle, W., Venturato, L., Griffiths, S., Grimbeek, P., McAllister, M., Oxlade, D. & Murfield, J. (2011b). Factors influencing quality of life for people with dementia: A qualitative perspective, *Aging and Mental Health*, 15(8), 970–7.

Nicholson, C. (2009). *Holding It Together: A Psycho-social Exploration of Living with Frailty in Old Age*. [Unpublished thesis]. London: Department of Adult Nursing, School of Community and Health Sciences, City University.

Preston, L., Marshall, A. & Bucks, R. (2007). Investigating the ways that older people cope with dementia: A qualitative study. *Aging & Mental Health*, 11, 131–43.

Rosenzweig, A. & Mishra, R. (2009). Evaluation and management of osteoporosis and fragility fractures in the elderly. *Aging Health*, 5(6), 833–50.

Sabat, S. (2001). *The Experience of Alzheimer's Disease. Life Through a Tangled Web*. Oxford: Blackwell Publishers.

Sarkisian, C., Shunkwiler, S., Aguilar, I. & Moore, A. (2006). Ethnic differences in expectations for ageing among older people. *The Journal of the American Geriatrics Society*, 54(8), 1277–82.

Statistics New Zealand. (2013). *National Population Estimates: At 30 June 2013*. Retrieved from http://www.statisphere.govt.nz

Strandberg, T., Pitkala, K., Tilvis, R., O'Neill, D. & Erkinjuntti, T. (2013). Geriatric syndromes – vascular disorders? *Annals of Medicine*, 45, 265–73.

Sykes, P. (2012). A best practice implementation project. *Journal of Nursing Care Quarterly*, 27(2), 146–53.

Tinetti, M., Inouye, S., Gill, T. & Doucette, J. (2005). Shared risk factors for falls, incontinence, and functional dependence. Unifying the approach to geriatric syndromes. *JAMA*, 273(3), 1348–53.

Tung, Y., Cooke, M. & Moyle, W. (2013). Sources older people draw on to nurture, strengthen and improve self-efficacy in managing rehabilitation following orthopaedic surgery. *Journal of Clinical Nursing*, 22(9–10), 1217–25.

Witucki Brown, J., Chen, S-I. Mitchell, C. & Province, A. (2007). Help-seeking by older husbands caring for wives with dementia. *Journal of Advanced Nursing*, 59, 352–60.

World Health Organization. (2012). *Dementia: A Public Health Priority*. Geneva.

7 Mental health and ageing

Wendy Moyle

Learning objectives

After reading this chapter you will be able to:

1 Describe social capital and the importance of social capital to mental ill health.

2 Describe the importance of culture and mental ill health.

3 Demonstrate an understanding of the common mental disorders in older age.

4 Demonstrate an understanding of the relationship of strengths-based nursing to the care of older people with mental disorders.

Introduction

This chapter focuses on the mental health of older people and provides an overview of mental disorders that are common in older age. The chapter also explores social capital, assessment and treatment of such disorders and the importance of culture and the strengths-based nursing approach to working with older adults with a mental disorder.

Social capital refers to 'social networks, social support, social cohesion, social participation, interpersonal trust and reciprocity' (Forsman, Nyqvist & Wahlbeck, 2011, p. 757). Social capital reflects an individual's relationships and their standing in their social community. The cognitive components of social capital that refer to an individual's social support and their perception of community have a close association with an individual's mental health. Where an older adult has high social support there is a negative association to mental ill health (Forsman, Nyqvist & Wahlbeck, 2011). One of the key roles of the nurse in practice is to ensure that the client has adequate social and physical support before they are discharged from any health practice setting. It is imperative that the nurse also understands the client's culture and the impact of this culture on their illness and support services.

> **Social capital**
> Reflects an individual's relationships and their standing in their social community.

Culture and mental health

Australia and New Zealand are culturally diverse countries. Both countries have relied on immigration to build their populations as fertility rates have declined over the last few decades. Furthermore, due to centuries of migration from the northern hemisphere, both countries also have minority indigenous populations. Australia and New Zealand have cultural diversity and rely on health professionals' practising **cultural safety**. In this sense cultural safety means that the client rather than the nurse or health practitioner defines if the care is safe. A culturally safe nurse is one who has undertaken a process of reflection on their own cultural identity and recognises the impact of the client's culture on their practice. Such a nurse recognises, respects and acknowledges the cultural rights of clients and allows the opportunity for them to direct care provision. Ball (2007, p. 1) describes five principles necessary for cultural safety:

Cultural safety
The client rather than the nurse or health practitioner defines if the care is safe.

- Protocols encouraging respect for cultural forms of engagement.
- Personal knowledge that allows an understanding of one's own cultural identity and sharing information about oneself to create a sense of equity and trust.
- Process of engaging in mutual learning, checking on cultural safety of the service recipient.
- Positive purpose ensuring the process yields the right outcome for the service recipient according to that recipient's values, preferences and lifestyle.
- Partnerships promoting collaborative practice.

As no culture is universal in practising person-centred care, a strengths-based approach will help to ensure older individuals and their needs are appropriately cared for.

Reflective activity

- Reflect upon and consider your cultural identity. What implications might your cultural identity have on your physical and mental illness?
- Reflect on traditional Aboriginal health models where all elements of life – physical, spiritual, moral, social and environmental – must balance to assist with health and well-being. What implications might such health beliefs have on physical and mental illness and care provision?

Mental health disorders in older adults

There are a number of conditions – such as depression, anxiety disorders, suicide, substance misuse, delirium, dementia and schizophrenia – which are common in older age; however these conditions do not occur *because* of ageing. Delirium and dementia have already been described in Chapter 6. You should refer back to this chapter for an overview of these disorders. The other common mental disorders in older age – depression, anxiety disorders, suicide, substance abuse and schizophrenia – will be explored in the sections that follow.

Depressive disorders

Depression is a common functional mental illness found in older people. Depressive disorders are known to be the leading cause of disability in the western world (World Health Organization, 2008) and can result in economic and social burden for families. Social burden affects in particular those living in the same household as being around people who are depressed can be challenging and can negatively influence the mood of the caregiver.

> **Depression**
> A state of low mood that has serious implications for physical and mental health.

Although depression is a common mental disorder it is not a normal part of ageing. It is thought that between 18 to 37 per cent of older people experience depression at some time in their later life (Ladin, 2008). However, this estimate is limited by the presentation of depression in older adults being difficult to diagnose when compared to younger adults. Older adults tend to focus their concerns on their physical symptoms and they often do not acknowledge that they feel sad or depressed when asked about their thoughts and feelings. This may be age related in that this group does not like to admit to not coping and saying they feel depressed suggests that they cannot cope with living in a fast, changing world. Older people tend to also feel there is a stigma associated with the discussion of mental health conditions. They may have a lack of understanding of the depressive disorder. Organisations such as the Black Dog Institute (www.blackdoginstitute.org.au) help both individuals and society by focusing on the education of society and in particular in the assessment, diagnosis and treatment of conditions such as depression. The aim of the Black Dog Institute is to remove the stigmatism about depression so that people are comfortable with seeking a diagnosis and can therefore be treated appropriately.

Symptoms of depression

Depression in older people affects mood, can lead to functional and cognitive decline (Steffens, 2009) and reduces quality of life (Chen et al., 2004). Symptoms of depression include:

- Cognitive changes such as slowing of memory.
- Diminished ability to think or concentrate.
- Indecisiveness, paranoia, agitation or retardation (being slowed down).
- Recurrent thoughts of death or suicide and persistent sadness lasting two or more weeks.
- Feelings of worthlessness, helplessness or inappropriate guilt.
- Physical symptoms such as muscle aches, abdominal pain, dry mouth, fatigue or loss of energy and headaches.
- Behavioural changes such as a change in appetite resulting in a significant decrease or increase in weight.
- Change in sleeping patterns.

Often these symptoms are attributed incorrectly to the older person having dementia or poor physical health. It is important therefore for society to understand that depression is not a normal part of ageing.

Types of depression

Melancholic depression is a severe biological form of depression in which the person experiences low energy, poor concentration, and slowed or agitated movements. This severe form is uncommon – it only affects 10 per cent of people with depression. The most common type of depression in older adults is non-melancholic or **major depression**, which is not biological but linked to acute or chronic stresses and to personality styles such as high anxiety levels, irritability indicating ongoing anxiety, low self-esteem and self-worth, self-imposed high standards, sensitivity to rejection, social avoidance, and a focus on one's own needs rather than on others'. The depression usually lifts when the stressful events are resolved. Depression is more common in older people when they have poor physical health and a history of depression in younger age. Unfortunately many of the medications used to treat physical symptoms common in older age such as hypertension, arthritis and pain, are associated with depression, raising the incidence of depression in older people (Chen et al., 2004).

Melancholic depression
A severe biological form of depression in which the person experiences low energy, poor concentration, and slowed or agitated movements.

Major depression
A depression that is not biological and is likely to be related to psychological causes such as stressful life events.

Assessment of depression

Early identification and treatment of depression and other mental conditions is critical in minimising functional decline in the older person and can contribute to a quicker recovery. Nurses have a role in the assessment of their older clients and the provision of a nursing care plan that takes into account their psychosocial situation and strengths. The nursing action is to send a powerful message to focus on the positive things in life rather than the negative problems as this can assist people's desire to live.

There are several instruments that can be used to help nurses assess older people for depression. The **Geriatric Depression Scale** (GDS) (Yesavage, Brink & Rose, 1983) is a well validated scale that assists in screening older people for depression. The GDS is available in many languages and is available in the public domain. The GDS can be downloaded from the following website: http://www.stanford. edu/%7Eyesavage/GDS.html. The GDS consists of 15 items and the person is asked to respond either 'yes' or 'no' to each question. Each item bolded in the scale scores one point and total scores greater than 5 suggest the presence of depression. Older people may suffer from depression, poor physical health and / or dementia concurrently and therefore it is important to take these factors into account during their assessment.

> **Geriatric Depression Scale** A well validated scale that assists in screening older people for depression.

Treatment of depression

Treatment of depression in older people can involve **cognitive behavioural therapy** (CBT) to help challenge negative thoughts, increase exercise and mental stimulation and encourage social activities. In more severe depression antidepressant medication is usually required. CBT is an individualised approach that helps the individual to learn or relearn healthier skills and habits. In cases of severe depression where the older person has not responded to antidepressant medication **electroconvulsive therapy** (ECT) may be used. ECT is administered while the person is under a general anaesthetic and given under the supervision of an anaesthetist, psychiatrist and nurse. An electric current is passed through the brain, intentionally inducing a brain seizure with the aim of reversing symptoms of mental illness. The risks of side effects are low when compared to the benefit individuals achieve particularly to those who have not responded to other treatments (Bebbington et al., 1980).

> **Cognitive behavioural therapy** An individualised approach that helps the individual to learn or relearn healthier skills and habits and to reduce negative thoughts.
>
> **Electroconvulsive therapy** A procedure that involves the passing of electric currents through the brain to trigger a seizure.

In addition older people need to be encouraged to take medication as prescribed, to eat a balanced diet, maintain regular exercise and sleep patterns, avoid illicit drugs and alcohol, maintain connections with family and friends, and facilitate a sense of achievement such as encouraging a role or responsibility that focuses on their strengths.

Factors associated with an improved chance of recovery from late life depression include: being female, being an extrovert, having no history of substance abuse, having no family history of depression, and, most importantly, having a high level of social support (Chen et al., 2004). When using a strengths-based care approach, these factors can be used to support the older person.

Rosie – ill health influence on diagnosis

Case scenario 7.1

Rosie is an 82 year old woman who was recently widowed following a happy marriage of almost 60 years. Rosie had cared for her husband John in their home for three years following his diagnosis with Alzheimer's disease. John had been difficult to care for – he was often very demanding and he constantly disturbed Rosie's sleep as he often woke during the early morning and demanded to go out of the house to work. Rosie was exhausted but reluctant to place John into a nursing home as she felt it was her duty to care for him at home. John died suddenly following complications from an infected mitral valve. Rosie's family believed that she would soon recover from her arduous caregiver role but they became concerned when, three months following John's death, she was still complaining of a lack of energy and no appetite. She had experienced significant weight loss. The family perceived that her symptoms were related to grief and loss and they did all they could to comfort her. As her weight continued to decline, the GP decided to start Rosie on antidepressants, although Rosie said she felt tired rather than sad.

Three months after commencement of antidepressant therapy the GP's practice nurse noticed that Rosie was continuing to decline and requested the GP to order a number of standard screening tests. The screening tests revealed that Rosie had breast cancer. Although Rosie's family were devastated to hear of her diagnosis, Rosie expressed relief as this provided her with a reason for her lack of energy. She confessed to the family that she believed she had become ill as her husband missed her and he was calling for her to come to him. Whilst she was interested to see him she said she was not ready to die as she had other people to live for such as her granddaughter's first child. Rosie decided she wanted to beat the cancer and was determined to have a mastectomy and radiation despite her family's belief that she was too frail to undergo such extensive surgery. The breast care nurse worked with Rosie's family to help them to recognise that Rosie had a right to make her own decision about her health care and treatment. Rosie survived the surgery and eight weeks later commenced radiotherapy.

Rosie was an inspiration to her family as well as to the staff who cared for her. She displayed strong courage throughout the multiple procedures she endured and whenever she felt low she recalled the things she enjoyed in life as these positive thoughts reminded her of the importance of living. Two years following surgery Rosie deteriorated and she was referred to a palliative care service. Rosie died two months later in a palliative care unit surrounded by the people she loved.

Reflective questions
Read and reflect on the case study of Rosie and address the following questions:

> Have you seen older people who have been diagnosed with depression that is secondary to a major physical condition?

> What was the GP practice nurse's role in Rosie's survival?

> What strengths did Rosie have that made her determined to survive?

> What might you do to help Rosie's family recognise that Rosie can be her own health care decision maker?

Anxiety and older adults

Anxiety disorders are common mental disorders associated with depression in later life but the more severe end of anxiety and depression is relatively rare in adults over 80 (Pachana et al., 2012). The DSM-IV (American Psychiatric Association, 2013) lists a number of anxiety disorders such as:

> **Anxiety disorder**
> A medical condition in which the individual suffers from persistent and excessive worry.

- Panic attack
- Acute stress disorder
- Agoraphobia
- Substance induced anxiety disorder
- Social anxiety disorder.
- Separation anxiety disorder.
- Selective mutism.

Anxiety is more common than depression in older people with phobias and is the most prevalent of the anxiety disorders (Blay & Marinho, 2012). Furthermore, the prevalence of anxiety and depression is more common in older people living in long-term care facilities (Smalbrugge et al., 2005). Anxiety can also accompany dementia. A recent survey found prevalence rates for anxiety in older people living in assisted living facilities in the US, with a diagnosis of dementia, were 11 to 18 per cent (Neville & Teri, 2011). Anxiety symptoms include:

- Nervousness
- Ruminations
- Irritability

- Inability to relax
- Hyper-vigilance, muscle tone or tension with associated aches and pains (American Psychiatric Association, 2000).

Anxiety disorders are persistent and can reduce a person's quality of life, especially if they cause avoidance of everyday activities or when the anxiety occurs in relation to activities such as leaving the home environment (Seignourel et al., 2008).

Neuroticism
A long-term tendency to be in a negative state.

Factors associated with the likelihood of anxiety or depression include greater **neuroticism**, poorer cognitive or physical function, greater disability and taking more medications (Gale et al., 2011). Therefore these factors increase the likelihood of older people being prone to anxiety disorders.

Assessment of anxiety

An instrument such as the **Geriatric Anxiety Inventory** (GAI) (Pachana et al., 2007) can help health professionals to assess the older person for anxiety. The GAI is a 20-item self-report or interviewer administered scale that measures anxiety in older people. The scale has good sensitivity and specificity in clinical and community samples (Pachana et al., 2007). The GAI is available free of charge to clinicians and academia from the GI website http://www.gai.net.au.

Geriatric Anxiety Inventory
A 20-item self-report or interviewer administered scale that measures anxiety in older people.

Rating Anxiety in Dementia (RAID) scale
A valid and reliable scale for measuring anxiety in people with dementia.

When older adults have dementia the **Rating Anxiety in Dementia (RAID) scale** (Shankar et al., 1999) can be used as it is more sensitive to changes in cognitive impairment as a result of the dementing disorder. The RAID has 18 items and has moderate to good reliability (Neville & Teri, 2011). The RAID is available from the following website: http://www.anxietydementia.co.uk/raid%20stuff.htm.

Treatment of anxiety

Pharmacological treatment using antidepressants or benzodiazepines is reported to have higher success rates in older people than psychological interventions (Blay & Marinho, 2012). However, treatment with benzodiazepines is often limited in older adults due to medication side effects such as risk for falls, fractures and cognitive impairment (Blay & Marinho, 2012). CBT has also been found to be effective for anxiety disorders in older adults (Gould, Coulson & Howard, 2012).

Suicide and older adults

At worst, a person with depression may attempt suicide (Chiu et al., 2004). Although **suicide** has been linked to depression, the majority of studies have been concerned with younger populations. Recent research however has demonstrated the risk of suicidal thoughts or suicidal risks in family carers of people living with dementia (O'Dwyer, Moyle & Wyk, 2013a; O'Dwyer et al., 2013b). Although carers are at increased risk of depression, this research reminds us that not all carers are depressed or succumb to suicidal thoughts. It seems that some carers may be resilient to the stressors of caregiving or they may recover quickly from the stressors. It is through the recognition of these qualities, the person's or the family's strengths, that nurses can make a difference to care through encouraging and empowering such strengths.

Suicide The act of intentionally causing one's own death.

Substance abuse

Alcohol misuse is common in older people followed by prescription drug misuse, although at much lower levels. In Australia it is reported that 15 per cent of older people consume alcohol daily and 5 per cent are at risk of short-term alcohol-related harm (Hunter & Lubman, 2010). Recent research has demonstrated a 10-fold increase in the odds for a suicide attempt in older adults with alcoholism (Morin et al., 2013). Individuals with long-term alcohol use are likely to experience a range of health problems including brain damage, liver failure, functional impairment, pancreatitis and increased risk of psychiatric and medical co-morbidity. The misuse of alcohol has enormous public health implications and early targeting and prevention of alcohol use disorder is important to reduce such health problems including suicide risk.

It is especially important for older people to understand that the ageing body responds differently to drugs and alcohol and that these changes are further compounded by their health as well as prescription and other over-the-counter medications.

Assessment and treatment of substance abuse

Early identification of substance abuse is recommended. The best way to identify alcohol misuse in older people is to ask questions about the amount and frequency of consumption and to consider the answers in relation to questions about the person's health and well-being. A simple screening tool such as theWorld Health Organization's Alcohol Use Disorders Identification Test (AUDIT) (Babor et al., 2001) will provide an indication of alcohol consumption in relation to consumption of standard drinks. AUDIT has three questions on drinking behaviour and dependence and four questions on the consequences of drinking. The current evidence suggests that older people with substance abuse problems are best supported through group therapies and self-help groups that emphasise social support (Cummings, Bride & Rawlins-Shaw, 2006). The AUDIT is freely available at the following website: http://www.sesml.org.au/uploads/all-documents/Mental_Health/Alcohol_Screen_AUDIT_Tool.pdf.

Schizophrenia and older adults

Schizophrenia is one of the most debilitating of the mental illnesses. Schizophrenia is usually considered to be an illness that affects young adults. However, this condition also occurs in older adults with the number being reported as one in seven patients (Vahia & Cohen, 2007). This number is expected to double within two decades alongside the ageing of the population (Vahia & Cohen, 2007). Schizophrenia is characterised by a breakdown in thinking and poor emotional responses. Common symptoms of schizophrenia include:

Schizophrenia
A mental disorder that is characterised by a breakdown in thinking and poor emotional responses.

- Delusions that are often bizarre
- Hallucinations such as hearing voices that are not there
- Disorganised speech (erratic or incoherent)
- Behavioural disturbance
- Negative symptoms (blunting of affect) (American Psychiatric Association, 2000).

A person must have at least two of these symptoms during a period of one month to be considered for a diagnosis of schizophrenia.

Schizophrenia is commonly seen as an illness of neurological functioning. While the exact cause of schizophrenia is not known there are genetic and environmental factors involved suggesting it is a disorder that has a complex interaction between these factors. People with a family history of schizophrenia are more at risk of developing it and environmental factors include drug use and prenatal stressors such as exposure to infection during gestation or birth (Mueser & Jeste, 2008).

Schizophrenia and strengths-based care

There are a limited number of studies that have investigated schizophrenia in older adults. A recent study from the Netherlands (Meesters et al., 2013) aimed to investigate the care needs of older people with schizophrenia. Of those patients aged 60 years and older, in contact with Dutch mental health services within a psychiatric catchment area, 114 patients with a mean age of 69 years (range 60–94 years) reported 7.6 needs of which 1.5 were unmet. The authors argue that the psychological and social needs appear to be under-serviced in this population and are associated with a reduced quality of life. Interestingly more than two thirds of the sample was women and the majority lived independently and alone. Their attendance at psychiatric services was fair to good. The inclusion of a strengths-based approach that takes into account patient needs and their perspective of quality of care are important in the delivery of quality comprehensive services. This is particularly important given the stigma associated with schizophrenia whereby society often judges these people as being unpredictable and dangerous to be around. In particular the opportunity for patients, staff and families to participate in community networking and for patients to tell their stories to others will help to reduce this stigmatisation.

Treatment of schizophrenia

Health promotion is especially important in people with schizophrenia, as the primary treatment is antipsychotic medication. Side effects include considerable weight gain, diabetes, Parkinsonian effects such as a blank, mask-like expression and salivary drooling, restless leg syndrome and motor rigidity.

CBT is also suited to individuals when they are in the well phase of their illness. The assumption is that CBT can positively influence symptoms by challenging behaviour and thinking.

Using a strengths-based approach – Judy

Judy is a 70 year old woman with a recent history reported by her family of unusual behaviour. She isolated herself in her room, stopped attending to her hygiene and expressed paranoid thoughts that her family were planning to kill her while she slept. Judy's family contacted her GP and, following a brief home visit where Judy refused to allow the GP into her room, she underwent an assessment by the crisis assessment and treatment team from the local hospital. Although cooperative during the assessment interview Judy appeared monosyllabic with slowed speech and energy. When asked if she was hearing voices Judy said she had and they were saying that her family wanted to get rid of her. The psychiatrist conducting the assessment made the diagnosis of schizophrenia. Judy began antipsychotic medication.

As she was not at risk, did not place her family at risk and her family were willing to look after her, Judy was cared for by community and home care services. The mental health nurse supported and educated Judy's family so that they could understand her illness and support her. Judy's family ensured that she was in a quiet and peaceful environment to help reduce any stimulation of delusional thinking. Judy had always enjoyed bush walking and so they introduced short walks in the garden and to a close by park as a means to assist her disordered thinking. Judy's family were strong in that they were united in their approach. They were willing to focus on Judy as the individual they knew rather than being solely concerned with her illness. They looked to the things Judy had always enjoyed and slowly reintroduced these back into her life. They accepted Judy's decisions in relation to the activities she wanted to participate in but they were also firm with her when at one stage she refused to take her prescribed medications. The family discussed with Judy the importance of the medication and they felt heartened by her response to continue taking it. With treatment and support Judy settled and continued to live with her family.

Reflective questions

Read and reflect on the case scenario of Judy and address the following questions:

> Have you come across an older person in your nursing practice with a diagnosis of schizophrenia? If so, what symptoms did this person display?

> What nursing interventions did the staff provide to help the person's symptoms?

> Were the person's family as helpful and understanding as Judy's family appears to be?

> What were Judy's family strengths and how did they use these to help her?

Strengths-based care approach to mental health care

A strengths-based care approach can assist an older person to improve their mood state to one that focuses on positive relationships and a will to live. A strengths-based care approach to help older people with mental health disorders should aim to focus on:

- Looking at what works when individuals are coping with their concerns and symptoms.
- Using an individual's strengths to build their confidence in dealing with their concerns and symptoms.
- Focusing on solutions rather than problems.
- Using positive language and focusing on hope for a positive future.
- Encouraging individuals to make plans and be involved in the decisions about their treatment and future path in collaboration with their nurse practitioner.

A strengths-based care approach focuses on and works with the individual. In this case study a client with mental ill health and her family's strengths promoted recovery from the illness and healing. Such an approach is of particular importance where clients feel stigmatised by their illness or where they feel they have a diseased body part and they may blame themselves for their illness. A strengths-based care approach can assist clients to feel empowered, to take control of their situation and to be the centre of the care and decision making process. Such an approach looks at what is working and functioning best for the client and helps them gain cultural identity and self-worth. This approach also enables a positive relationship between the client and nurse and helps to reduce any self-doubts that client may have.

The nurse is encouraged to use the ROPES Assessment (see Chapter 3) to assess emotional and behavioural health of the client and their family, as well as their competencies and characteristics. Such a focus can support the construction of solutions rather than focus on the client's problems. Where clients have a strong cultural identity it is also important to link them with culturally specific services. For example, the indigenous psychological services are the only provider of psychology specific services for indigenous people in Australia (http://indigenouspsychservices.com.au). Such a service has developed culturally specific assessment tools, workforce training programs to determine and improve competencies unique to indigenous people, as well as community intervention programs.

Summary

- Cultural diversity relies on health professionals practising cultural safety whereby the client defines if the care provided is safe.
- A culturally safe practitioner is one who has undertaken a process of reflection on their own cultural identity and recognises the impact of the client's culture on their practice.

- Where an individual has strong relationships within their community that may, for example, be built on their position within the community this may protect them from mental illness.
- The common mental disorders in older age include depression, anxiety disorders, substance abuse and schizophrenia and these conditions may lead the person to attempt suicide.
- A strengths-based nursing approach to care for older people with mental disorders takes into account factors that may improve the chance of recovery from mental ill health.

Conclusion

This chapter examined the topic of mental ill health in older adults and highlighted common instruments to help with its assessment and common treatments. The chapter provides several case studies that can be used to help readers understand the impact of mental ill health on older adults as well as those caring for them. A strengths-based approach to nursing care may help older people with mental disorders improve their self-worth and reduce or prevent psychosocial problems that they may have.

Further reading

You may like to take a look at the following reading recommendations:

- 'mindhealthconnect' – this outlines resources from leading health organisations in Australia and focuses on mental health disorders of older people. It can be found at the following website: http://www.mindhealthconnect.org.au
- An excellent overview of Maori mental health resources is available at: http://www.mentalhealth.org.nz/page/191-maori-mental-health
- For an overview of indigenous social and emotional well-being for people working, studying or interested in this issue: http://www.healthinfonet.ecu.edu.au

References

American Psychiatric Association. (2013). *Diagnostic and Statistical Manual of Mental Disorders*. (5th edition). Arlington, VA.

Babor, T., Higgins-Biddle, J., Saunders, J. & Monteiro, M. (2001). *AUDIT: The Alcohol Use Disorders Identification Test. Guidelines for Use in Primary Care*. Geneva: Department of Mental Health and Substance Dependence, World Health Organization.

Ball, J. (2007). Supporting Aboriginal Children's Development. *In Early Childhood Development Intercultural Partnerships*, Melbourne: University of Victoria. Retrieved from http://www.ecdip.org/capacity/

Bebbington, P., Bennett, D., Birley, J., Clare, A., Cutting, J., Kumar, R., . . . Williams, P. (1980). ECT: Balancing risks and benefits. *British Medical Journal*, 280(6216), 792.

Blay, S. & Marinho, V. (2012). Anxiety disorders in old age. *Current Opinion in Psychiatry*, 25, 462–7.

Chen, R., Hu, Z., Qin, Z., Xu, X. & Copeland, J. (2004). A community-based study of depression in older people in Hefei China-the GMS-AGECAT prevalence, case validation and socio-economic correlates. *International Journal Geriatric Psychiatry*, 19, 407–13.

Chiu, H., Yip, P., Chi, I., Chan, S., Tsoh, J., Kwan, C., . . . Caine, E. (2004). Elderly suicide in Hong Kong: A case-controlled psychological autopsy study. *Acta Psychiatrica Scandinavica*, 109, 299–305.

Cummings, S., Bride, B. & Rawlins-Shaw, A. (2006). Alcohol abuse treatment for older adults – a review of recent empirical research. *Journal of Evidence-Based Social Work*, 3(1), 79–99.

Forsman, A., Nyqvist, F. & Wahlbeck, K. (2011). Cognitive components of social capital and mental health status among older adults: A population based cross-sectional study. *Scandinavian Journal of Public Health*, 39, 757–65.

Gale, C., Sayer, A., Cooper, C., Dennison, E., Starr, J., Whalley, L., . . . Deary, I. (2011). Factors associated with symptoms of anxiety and depression in five cohorts of community-based older people: The HALCyon (Healthy Ageing across the Life Course) Program. *Psychological Medicine*, 41, 2057–73.

Gould, R., Coulson, M. & Howard, R. (2012). Efficacy of cognitive behavioural therapy for anxiety disorders in older people: A meta-analysis and meta-regression of randomized controlled trials. *Journal American Geriatric Society*, 60, 218–29.

Hunter, B. & Lubman, D. (2010). Substance misuse: Management in the older population. *Australian Family Physician*, 39(10), 738–41.

Ladin, K. (2008). Risk of late-life depression across 10 European Union countries: Deconstructing the education effect. *Journal Aging Health*, 20, 653–70.

Meesters, P., Comijs, H., Droes, R., de Haan, L., Smit, J., Eikelenboom, P., . . . Stek, M. (2013). The care needs of elderly patients with schizophrenia spectrum disorders. *The American Journal of Geriatric Psychiatry*, 21, 129–37.

Morin, J., Wiktorsson, S., Marlow, T., Olesen, P., Skoog, I. & Waern, M. (2013). Alcohol use disorder in elderly suicide attempters: A comparison study. *The American Journal of Geriatric Psychiatry*, 21, 196–203.

Mueser, K. & Jeste, D. (2008). *Clinical Handbook of Schizophrenia*. New York: Guilford Press.

Neville, C. & Teri, L. (2011). Anxiety, anxiety symptoms, and associations among older people with dementia in assisted-living facilities. *International Journal of Mental Health Nursing*, 20, 195–201.

O'Dwyer, S., Moyle, W. & van Wyk, S. (2013a). Suicidal ideation and resilience in family carers of people with dementia: A qualitative study, *Aging and Mental Health*, 17(6), 753–60.

O'Dwyer, S., Moyle, W., Zimmer-Gembeck, M. & De Leo, D. (2013b). Suicidal ideation in family carers of people with dementia: A pilot study. *International Journal of Geriatric Psychiatry.* doi:10.1002/gps.3941

Pachana, N., Byrne, G., Siddle, H., Koloski, N., Harley, E. & Arnold, E. (2007). Development and validation of the Geriatric Anxiety Inventory. *International Psychogeriatrics*, 19, 103–14. doi:10.1017/S1041610206003504

Pachana, N., McLaughlin, D., Leung, J., Byrne, G. & Dobson, A. (2012). Anxiety and depression in adults in their eighties: Do gender differences remain? *International Psychogeriatrics*, 24, 145–50.

Seignourel, P., Kunik, M., Snow, L., Wilson, N. & Stanley, M. (2008). Anxiety in dementia: A critical review. *Clinical Psychology Review*, 28, 1071–82.

Shankar, K., Walker, M., Frost, D. & Orrell, M. (1999). The development of a valid and reliable scale for rating anxiety in dementia (RAID). *Aging and Mental Health*, 3, 39–49.

Smalbrugge, M., Jongenelis, L., Pot, A.M., Beekman, A.T. & Eefsting, J.A. (2005). Comorbidity of anxiety and depression in nursing home patients. *International Journal of Geriatric Psychiatry*, 20, 218–26. doi: 10.1002/gps.1269

Steffens, D.C. (2009). A multiplicity of approaches to characterize geriatric depression and its outcomes. *Current Opinion in Psychiatry*, 22, 522–6.

Vahia, I. & Cohen, C. (2007). Psychosocial interventions and successful aging: New paradigms for improving outcome for older schizophrenia patients. *American Journal of Psychiatry*, 15, 987–90.

World Health Organization. (2008). *Global Burden of Disease. 2004 Update.* Geneva. Retrieved from http://www.who.int/healthinfo/global_burden_disease/ projections/ en/index.html

Yesavage, J., Brink, T. & Rose, T. (1983). Development and validation of a geriatric depression rating scale: A preliminary report. *Journal of Psychiatric Research*, 17, 27.

8

The role of the family in care of older people

Wendy Moyle and Marguerite Bramble

Learning objectives

After reading this chapter you will be able to:

1. Describe the caregiving roles family members play in care of older people who require long-term care.

2. Outline the positive and negative psychosocial impacts of this role.

3. Describe respite care in relation to family caregiving.

4. Describe Consumer Directed Care and the positive influencers of this.

5. Identify evidence-based nursing interventions for family caregivers, including Family Involvement in Care, an intervention for people with dementia and their families.

Introduction

This chapter focuses on the role of family members in care of older people and in this context the term **family caregiver** will be used. A family caregiver is someone, such as a family member, friend or neighbour, excluding paid or volunteer carers organised by formal services, who has been identified as providing regular and sustained **informal care** and assistance to the client without payment other than a pension or benefit. With the ageing population and the rising prevalence of chronic disease there is an increasing requirement from health service providers for more involvement from family caregivers to assist in providing care and support to those in need. This involvement may be on a number of levels, from being responsible for coordinating primary caregiving in the home environment to providing support to formal carers in long-term care. The opportunities and encouragement given to family members to be involved in the care of the resident in long-term care

> **Family caregiver**
> An unpaid caregiver (family, friend or neighbour) who provides care, in a voluntary capacity, for another's physical, emotional and developmental well-being.

> **Informal care**
> Regular, sustained care to a person in need of support on an unpaid basis.

is essential to the provision of quality of care. Such opportunities are not without challenges and the problems of implementing a family involvement in care focus within long-term care will be discussed later in the chapter.

A tradition of family caregiving

Historically families worldwide have played a role in providing care, either to children, spouses or parents, across the lifespan. In Australia and New Zealand, governments and health services are responding to the need and desire for older people to be cared for in their homes for as long as possible by providing an increased range of case managed Primary Health Care and Home Care Packages, described in more detail in Chapter 4 (Australian Government Department of Health and Ageing, 2010; King, 2001). As discussed in Chapters 4 and 5 gerontological nurses can play a vital role as case managers and care coordinators in providing support to family caregivers as well as clients as they navigate their way through the range of services available (Rees, 2013). Even with the increasing availability of aged community services family and friends will continue to provide 80 to 90 per cent of the care to older adults at home (Hunter, 2012). It is important that nurses in practice understand that from a consumer perspective family caregivers seek access to quality community care and support-based on evidence-based practice.

Family caregiving in New Zealand

In New Zealand family informal care is defined as help or support provided by a family member, friend or neighbour to a disabled, sick or frail person (Statistics New Zealand, 2006). Informal carers are typically unpaid, although in some cases may be paid (New Zealand Department of Labour, 2011). In 2006 an estimated 30 600 disabled adults aged 65 and over with high support needs were living in households rather than in long-term care. This included 14 900 (49%) living in couple only households and 4700 (15%) living by themselves. From 2001 to 2006 the proportion of older unpaid carers grew at a faster rate than the general population, and female caregivers outnumbered male carers in every age group. By ethnicity, female Maori were most likely to be caregivers, followed closely by female Maori/Europeans (Statistics New Zealand, 2006).

In New Zealand 'ageing' was described as the most common cause of disability for adults aged 65 years and over, affecting more than half of adults with a recognised disability (Statistics New Zealand, 2006). Disease or illness was the second most common cause for this age group (47% of adults with disability). In 2008 the

New Zealand Carers' Strategy and Five-year Action Plan was developed with the aim to promote greater recognition and understanding of the needs of individuals, families/whanau/aiga who care for and support people who need help with their everyday living. The strategy also aims to ensure that family carers have choices and opportunities to participate in family life, social activities, employment and education, and that carers' voices are heard in decision making that affects them (Ministry of Social Development New Zealand, 2013).

Family caregiving in Australia

In Australia family caregivers are described as primary or non-primary carers (Australian Bureau of Statistics, 2012). A primary carer is described as a person aged 15 years and over who provides the most informal assistance with core activities (communication, mobility and self-care) to a person with a disability or to a person aged 65 years or over (Australian Bureau of Statistics, 2012).

According to the most recent data from the Australian Bureau of Statistics (ABS), in 2012 there were 2.7 million people in Australia who were providing informal care as a primary carer to an older person or someone with a disability or long-term health condition. One in five (540 000) of primary carers were aged 65 years or more and caring for a partner. Of those primary carers whose main recipient was a parent, most were aged 45 to 64 years (378 000). The majority of primary carers (83%) resided in the same household as the person for whom they provided the most care. Of those primary carers whose main recipient of care did not live with them, most were caring for a parent (67% or around 86 900 primary carers).

In 2012 females made up the majority of family caregivers, representing 70 per cent of primary carers and 56 per cent of carers overall. There were similar proportions of male and female non-primary caregivers (49% and 51% respectively). Among people aged 55 to 64 years, there were 126 700 female primary carers (9.6%) and 90 900 male primary carers (4.7%). There were almost equal numbers of male and female primary carers in the 75 years and over age group (an estimated 35 100 males and 36 500 females). It is interesting to note that after the age of 65 years, the proportion of female carers declined, whereas the proportion of male carers continued to increase. This was the case for both primary carers and non-primary carers (Australian Bureau of Statistics, 2012). From the age of 75 years there were almost double the proportion of male non-primary carers compared with female non-primary carers (15.8% of males compared with 8.5% of females). This equated to around 91 000 male and 61 500 female, non-primary carers.

Of the many reasons primary caregivers in Australia reported for taking on the role of the main informal care provider, the most common was a sense of family responsibility (63%). The next most common reason was a feeling that they could provide better care than anybody else (50%), followed by a feeling of emotional obligation to undertake the role (41%). When the person being cared for was older it was more likely that no other friends or family were available to take on the caring role (32% compared with 22% for recipients aged less than 64 years) (Australian Bureau of Statistics, 2012).

The ABS (2012) reported that of the population of older Australians with a disability, most lived in a private dwelling (85%) and needed some form of assistance (56%) with one or more activities of daily life. While the majority of older people with a disability lived with others, there were around 61 300 with a profound core activity limitation living alone in a private dwelling in 2012. In 2012, 87 per cent of older Australians reported having a long-term health condition. Of the 2.8 million older people who reported a long-term health condition, 93 per cent were most affected by a physical condition, while 7 per cent said a mental or behavioural disorder caused them the most problems. Considering all people aged 65 years or more, the most frequently reported health conditions were arthritis (16%), hypertension (11%) and back problems (9%). Dementia or Alzheimer's disease (2.7%) was the most frequently reported condition relating to a mental or behavioural disorder.

Futhermore, the ABS (2012) stated that the prevalence of some health conditions varies with age. For example, in 2012, a person aged 80 years or over was seven times more likely to identify dementia or Alzheimer's disease as their main long-term health condition than someone aged 65 to 79 years (7.6% compared with 1.0%). In contrast, the proportion of those who reported arthritis as their main condition was similar across these age groups (17.3% compared with 15.9%). In 2012, around 1.4 million older people needed assistance with at least one activity because of disability or age (42%). Assistance was most commonly needed for health care tasks (25%) and property maintenance (23%). The need for assistance for older persons differed between the genders, with almost half of older females (49%) reporting a need for assistance with at least one activity, compared with around a third of older males (34%). Females were more likely than males to have needed assistance with household chores (23% compared with 12%), mobility (21% compared with 14%) and transport (20% compared with 14%). Of those who needed assistance, the common informal providers were their spouse or partner (34%) or their daughter (22%). Common formal sources were private commercial organisations (37%) and government organisations (30%).

The Australian data from the ABS provides an opportunity for nurses in practice to examine the latest trends in carer demographics, including changes related to family caregiving and the carer–recipient relationship. The statistics also allow for comparison of the experiences of carers of people with different disabling conditions, for example chronic obstructive pulmonary disease (COPD) and dementia, and an understanding of family caregivers' evolving needs based on the characteristics of the recipients of their care. The needs of couples with dementia, for example, are likely to be different from the needs of a couple dealing with the aftermath of a stroke or a heart attack. Similarly the needs of filial family caregivers who care for older people with chronic illness also differ from those of spouses or friends of the same age.

In primary care the role of family caregivers takes on 'strategic importance' in designing services so that older people can stay at home for as long as possible (Nolan et al., 2003, p. 1). This means moving beyond considering the responsibilities of caring as simply a source of burden and stress and considering more innovative, holistic and dynamic approaches to support family caregiving.

Family caregiving roles are being more clearly acknowledged in the latest round of economic reforms such as the Living Longer Living Better aged care reforms. As part of these reforms the Australian government is expanding home care to assist people to remain at home as long as possible so they have delivered choice and flexibility for people living at home through the development of Consumer Directed Care (CDC). This concept was first introduced in Chapter 4 and will be discussed in more detail later in this chapter.

Up until now this chapter has predominantly concentrated broadly on family caregiving and caregiving in the home. The chapter will now change the focus to consider family caregivers within the context of long-term care. While long-term care placement is challenging for a family to consider it does not necessarily reduce caregiver distress (Moyle, Edwards & Clinton, 2002).

Working with family caregivers in long-term care

As indicated earlier, encouraging the role of the family caregiver in the context of long-term care is fraught with many challenges. An initial challenge is the fact that some family members do not participate in the care of their older family member once placed within long-term care. Some of the reasons for this include a lack of knowledge of how they might contribute once they are no longer primarily responsible for the care of their family member, and fears and concerns about watching their family member deteriorate (Moyle, Edwards & Clinton, 2002). Furthermore, when there are different views between family and staff on quality of care and quality of life this can add to the barrier between staff and family and result in family further limiting their role. At the heart of this debate is the tension between the opportunities for enhancing the life of a person with a chronic condition such as dementia and the practicalities of the environment, in particular, staffing levels (Moyle, 2010; Moyle et al., 2011).

The dynamic interplay between the difficulties, satisfactions and coping strategies of family caregivers is complex and changing. The needs of family caregivers change over time, depending on the nature of the disease process. It is important that nurses, as part of the multidisciplinary team, take this into consideration when identifying the support systems required (Bulechek et al., 2013). While many family members may be in the ideal position to maintain the resident's link to the outside world and in particular to their social networks, staff must establish and maintain relationships with family members and provide them with support. As family caregivers become more experienced in their role, nurses can build on a relationship-centred approach to family care (Nolan et al., 2003). One way of achieving more formal relationships is by establishing **partnership models** for clients, families and staff across settings (Bramble, Moyle & Shum, 2011; Nolan, Bauer & Nay 2009). A partnership model views the family as diverse people with their own individual needs for support and a potential resource for improving quality of care of the resident/client. Such an approach has similarities to the strengths-based approach that moves the focus of care away from tasks and problems to seeing the person and their abilities. As outlined in Chapter 3 the focus in a strengths-based approach is on the strengths of the person and family, to identify the strengths and to use the strengths that are available to them. Rather than being an expert the nurse's role in this position is to empower people to take the lead in their care and care decisions.

Partnership models Derive from the view that families themselves are clients and a potential resource for improving quality of care for the resident with dementia.

Relational approach

It is also important that nurses develop a **relational approach** with family caregivers that reaches across health settings, involves family caregivers in a participatory role and can provide appropriate support as needs change (Nolan

et al., 2003). Establishing the importance of relationships in providing care may benefit the caregiver or the person in receipt of care.
Relationship-centred care is discussed in more detail in Chapter 3.

> **Relational approach** Refers to the importance of relationships in providing care.

Initially many family caregivers are not aware of the services
that are available from health care providers in their communities.
This particularly applies to people from other countries, cultures and indigenous people. Educating family caregivers is a critical role of nurses and em-
powers them to be more proactive with health care providers. Although the
majority of family caregivers enjoy the opportunity to care for their family, the
work is demanding and tiring. Respite care may help family caregivers have a
break from their caregiving role.

Respite care in Australia

Substantial resources have been provided to help family caregivers provide
community care and to also aid them in taking leave from the burden of care.
In Australia respite care can be provided for a few hours or a few days, or for a
short period of time if, for example, the family caregiver is recovering from an
illness. Respite care can be provided in the care recipient's home for a few hours
to overnight care; in a day centre for a full or half a day of care; in a respite cottage for overnight or weekend care, in residential care for one to six weeks, or if
required in emergency care at times of an unforeseen event. In Australia funding for such services is from the National Respite for Carers Program (NRCP)
and Home and Community Care Program (HACC). The Australian government pays for the majority of the respite care, but it is expected that family will
contribute to the cost if they can afford to do so. Different fee structures are in
place for the different types of respite services available.

Although respite services have been in place for some years the uptake of
respite care has not met government expectations. Stockwell-Smith and colleagues (2010) interviewed family caregivers who were not currently using respite services in an attempt to identify some of the reasons for the poor uptake.
They found that family caregivers held the role of care of the recipient as central and they did not feel they could easily relinquish it to a service provider.
Furthermore, the family caregivers discussed their frustrations at not being
able to decipher and negotiate the service provisions. So it was difficult for family caregivers to even understand the available services.

A strengths-based approach in this situation would be to empower the family and client to take the lead in their care and respite requirements and to work

in collaboration with health care providers. The nurse would encourage the family caregiver to outline the care provisions they would like to see continue into respite care, to tell their stories about the areas of care they enjoy the most, and the opportunities they would like put into place so that they can see that their needs, as well as the needs of the care recipient, are being met. Such an arrangement will enable the family caregiver to recognise their important role in the care provision of their family member.

Respite care in New Zealand

The New Zealand Ministry of Health provides community-based services to provide breaks for the carers of a disabled person. Respite care is usually short-term and intermittent. The Needs Assessment and Service Coordination (NASC) organisation provides the service when a family caregiver/whanau requires a short-term break from their caregiving role. The amount of funded respite support is based on the needs and availability of services.

Consumer Directed Care

To help support family and older people, in addition to respite services the Australian government has recently introduced CDC. CDC allows the delivery of care where carers and consumers can have a greater control over the types of care and services they wish to access and the delivery of those services. CDC aligns well to a strengths-based approach in that it assumes the care recipient and the family caregiver will do better when they are helped to identify and to use their strengths and resources around them. CDC operation is based on six principles:

- *Consumer choice and control:* to access information and to build a package that supports them to live life as they want.
- *Rights:* CDC should acknowledge the rights of an older person.
- *A respectful and balanced partnership* between consumers and home care providers.
- *Participation:* community and civic participation.
- *Wellness and reablement:* CDC packages should be offered within a restorative or reablement framework.
- *Transparency:* older people have the right to use their budgets to purchase services they choose and need to have access to information that will allow them to decide on how their funding might be spent.

Although CDC is in its infancy in Australia it has been in practice in the UK in both disability and care services for a longer period of time. Escalating health costs and rising unmet needs of clients are two of the drivers of the CDC approach where funds are allocated to trusts or to individual budgets. The key benefits of CDC are the responsiveness to individual requirements and that the approach offers the client more bargaining power with service providers.

In Australia all new Home Care Packages from 1 August 2013 are delivered on a CDC basis and from July 2015 all packages of care will operate on a CDC basis. A CDC agreement is made between the care recipient and the provider of care about the services that will be received and their cost. The aim is for the care provider to develop a care package that is based on the needs of and agreed by the care recipient. Under such arrangements any government funding received by the care recipient will be paid directly to the provider who can spend the funds only on the items of services agreed upon.

Measuring well-being of family caregivers: a strengths-based approach

For older adults with chronic conditions such as cancer, heart and lung disease, and dementia, caregiving can extend and evolve gradually over a period of years. During that time there is usually a need for more intense medical care or rehabilitation services. It is during these times that nurses should assess family caregiver well-being and observe for signs of caregiver burden. Caregiver burden is described as the extent to which family caregivers perceive their emotional or physical health, social life and financial status has suffered as a result of caring for their relative (Bramble, 2009; Bramble, Moyle & Shum, 2011). Specific functional consequences of caregiver burden include depression, disturbed sleep, social isolation, poor physical health and feelings of anger, guilt, grief, anxiety, hopelessness and helplessness (Bramble, 2009; Bramble, Moyle & McAllister, 2009).

Family caregivers provide care for several reasons such as a sense of love or reciprocity, spiritual fulfilment, or a sense of duty. Although the negative aspects of caregiving appear to receive the most attention, caregiving also brings with it positive feelings and outcomes such as the enjoyment felt from being with the person being cared for, a reciprocal bond, feelings of accomplishment and increased faith. In the UK and the US there has been a move away from simply reducing carer stress to enriching relationships and developing theoretically based interventions that are meaningful for carers and are based on their knowledge and 'expertise' (Bulechek et al., 2013; Rees, 2013). Other factors that influence the experience of being a caregiver are cultural influences, the nature of the illness and other family supports. Nurses can build on these positive aspects of caring by identifying strengths in providing support through case managed care options, education and therapeutic nursing interventions. An example of nursing interventions for family caregivers is presented in Table 8.1.

TABLE 8.1 *Nursing outcomes and nursing interventions for promoting wellness in family caregivers*

TYPE OF NEED	NURSING OUTCOMES	NURSING INTERVENTIONS
Needs related to caregiver role	Caregiver emotional/physical health	Caregiver support
	Caregiver well-being	Case management
	Caregiver stressors	Family support
	Caregiver home care readiness	Resiliency promotion
	Caregiver–recipient relationship	Role enhancement
	Caregiver adaptation	Self-awareness enhancement
	To institutionalisation	Support groups
Needs related to using resources and managing care	Information processing	Decision making support
	Knowledge	Health education
	Health resources	Health system guidance
	Participation in health care decisions	Referral
	Role performance	Respite care
		Support system enhancement
		Teaching
Psychosocial needs	Anxiety level	Active listening
	Coping, depression level	Anticipatory guidance
	Family coping	Anxiety reduction
	Family resilience	Emotional support
	Fear level	Grief work facilitation
	Grief resolution	Other therapies
	Loneliness, stress	
Spiritual and quality of life needs	Hope	Spiritual support
	Leisure participation	Guilt work facilitation
	Quality of life	Sleep enhancement
	Sleep	
	Social involvement and support	
	Spiritual health	

Source: Adapted from Hunter, 2012, p. 556

strengths-based approach to family caregiving

You are working as a nurse graduate in a community setting in an urban suburb. You have been asked by the local community nursing service to visit an 83 year old Italian man, Carlos, who has been caring for his 81 year old wife, Bella since her osteoporosis and ischaemic heart disease severely impacted on her ability to function three years ago. You note when you read Carlos and Bella's care plans that Carlos has recently been showing signs of anxiety and loneliness and is finding it increasingly difficult to cope in the caregiving role. He has stated that he feels he is unable to take Bella to their beloved Italian community church once a week, or to leave her to attend on his own. He receives care assistance with meal preparation, cleaning and shopping.

When you arrive at Carlos and Bella's home at 9 am you find Bella still in bed and Carlos sitting on the side of the bed holding her hand. You note that the kitchen has not been cleaned for days and the bathroom also requires attention. You ask permission to sit with them and begin your assessment, based on the information provided by the community nursing service as well as your observations.

Reflective questions

Read and reflect on the above case study and address the following questions:

› Using a strengths-based approach what initial information would you be most interested in gaining from Carlos and Bella?

› After your initial conversation with Carlos and Bella you find that their major support, their daughter Francine, has returned to their home country for 12 months. Their son Bruce lives 120 km away on a farm. In consideration of Carlos' family caregiving role and the characteristics of Bella's condition, what strategies would you develop with them to ensure their short-term and long-term needs are met?

› What other health professionals and health services would you contact to provide for the functional needs of Carlos and Bella?

› What other social or spiritual supports would you initiate to provide for Carlos' psychosocial and spiritual needs?

Family caregiving of people with dementia

In Australia and New Zealand development of models of family caregiving for people with dementia continues to lag behind the UK and the US (Bauer, 2006; Bauer & Nay, 2003; Kellett, 2007). In both the UK and the US the notion of partnership between families and staff has derived from the view that families themselves are clients and a potential resource for improving quality of care of the resident with dementia (Maas et al., 1994; Maas et al., 2004; Nolan, Bauer & Nay, 2009b; Nolan et al., 2004). As the person with dementia's cognitive capacity and level of engagement deteriorates, it is the family caregiver who then becomes the 'surrogate client', and their involvement in the daily therapeutic practice of nurses provides a vital resource for understanding their relative's individual care needs (Bramble, Moyle & Shum, 2011).

Dementia and family caregiving: the role of the nurse in practice

When a family member reports that an older person's behaviour or attitude has changed it is important to acknowledge and document this information. Family caregivers often notice subtle changes weeks or months before they become apparent to health professionals (Tabloski, 2010). As the dementia develops family caregivers become surrogate decision makers and make judgements and decisions based on their intimate knowledge of the person with dementia, their preferences and quality of life (Tabloski, 2010). The nurse's scope of practice in this case is to ensure that the rights of family caregivers, as well as the person with dementia, are upheld. This applies particularly in the later stages of the illness and will be further discussed in Chapter 10.

The following section highlights a successful partnership intervention called the Family Involvement in Care.

The Family Involvement in Care intervention

Family Involvement in Care (FIC) intervention
Derived from evidence that working partnerships based on knowledge exchange and negotiation of roles can improve well-being for staff, families and people with dementia.

The **Family Involvement in Care (FIC) intervention** was developed in the US by Professor Meridean Maas and has been added to the Nursing Interventions Classification (NIC) as a standardised intervention (Bulechek et al., 2013). The FIC intervention was derived from evidence that working partnerships based on knowledge exchange and negotiation of roles can improve well-being for staff, families and people with dementia (Maas et al., 2004). The FIC model underwent extensive trialling with the intervention results indicating that the FIC intervention in particular improves the caregiving experience of family members in long-term care as well as staff attitudes towards family members.

In Australia a partial replication of the FIC model was explored using a mixed-method approach in residential dementia care (Bramble et al., 2009; Bramble, Moyle & Shum, 2011). The partnership is based on the premise that the family caregivers are clients and a valuable resource for improving quality of care for the person with dementia. The research found that caregiving arrangements between staff and family improved as did the care for the person living with dementia (Bramble et al., 2009; Bramble, Moyle & Shum, 2011).

mily Involvement in Care (FIC)

Case scenario 8.2

Bill is an 87 year old ex-engineer who was diagnosed with vascular dementia six years ago. When his wife passed away five years ago it became clear to his two daughters that Bill could not care for himself at home. He agreed to move into a long-term care facility that was within easy travelling distance of one of his daughters. Both daughters were keen to be involved in Bill's care and care decisions and readily agreed to become involved in an FIC approach to care. Bill's daughters were educated about FIC and provided with a manual showing opportunities where they might like to become involved in his care.

The registered nurse met the daughters and planned their involvement and evaluation of the involvement with them. One daughter contracted to visit three times a week during lunch meals so that she could help and encourage Bill to eat as he has recently lost his appetite and had been losing weight. The second daughter contracted to visit three times a week to read to Bill as his failing eyesight had reduced his opportunity to read and reading had always been one of his pleasures in life. The daughters asked the care staff to take Bill to a small lounge in the facility each afternoon where he could

enjoy a view of the garden, an activity he had enjoyed in his later life, and would give him an opportunity to chat with other residents.

After one month the registered nurse, the daughters and Bill met to discuss progress to date. Bill expressed that he was delighted to see his daughters and he very much enjoyed the visit each afternoon to the quiet lounge. The daughters described that they felt valued by the staff by being given the opportunity for involvement in Bill's care and the registered nurse explained that she and her team had learnt a lot more about Bill's social biography during their taking of Bill to the quiet lounge each afternoon. Bill's moods improved and he had put on weight.

Reflective questions
Read the case scenario of Bill and address the following questions:

> What might have been some of the key factors in the success of the family and staff engagement in Bill's care?

> What are some of the benefits of the FIC approach?

> How might you encourage family and staff to work together towards a mutual benefit to the resident?

Summary

- Family caregiving roles are important in the care of older people who require long-term care.
- Although there is an emphasis on the negative aspects of family caregiving there are a number of positive implications that are beneficial to both the caregiver and the recipient of care.
- Although Consumer Directed Care is in its infancy in Australia it has been found to have a positive influence on quality of care and quality of life of the care recipient.
- The Family Involvement in Care Partnership intervention has been shown to be a successful intervention with positive outcomes for all involved.

Conclusion

This chapter examined the topic of family involvement in care of older people across settings. The chapter outlines the importance of the demographics of family caregivers in understanding their needs. A strengths-based approach to care alongside evidence-based interventions will encourage the care recipient and caregiver to become partners in the care.

Further reading

You may like to take a look at the following reading recommendations:

- The following website, which provides examples from the Victorian Government, Australia on involving families in the care of people living with dementia: http://www.health.vic.gov.au/dementia/changes/family.htm
- For more information about Consumer Directed Care visit: http://www.livinglongerlivingbetter.gov.au/internet/living/publishing.nsf/Content/Consumer-Directed-Care-Home-Care-Packages

References

Australian Bureau of Statistics. (2012). *Disability, Ageing and Carers, Australia: Summary of Findings*. Canberra.

Australian Government Department of Health and Ageing. (2010). *Building a 21st Century Primary Health Care System: Australia's First National Primary Health Care Strategy*. Canberra.

Bauer, M. (2006). Collaboration and control: Nurses' constructions of the role of family in nursing home care. *Journal of Advanced Nursing*, 54(1), 45–52.

Bauer, M. & Nay, R. (2003). Family and staff partnerships in long-term care. A review of the literature. *Journal of Gerontological Nursing*, 29(10), 46.

Bramble, M. (2009). *Promoting Family Involvement in Residential Dementia Care: An Education Intervention*. [Unpublished doctoral dissertation]. Brisbane: Griffith University.

Bramble, M., Moyle, W. & McAllister, M. (2009). Seeking connection: Family care experiences following long-term dementia care placement. *Journal of Clinical Nursing*, 18, 3118–25.

Bramble, M., Moyle, W. & Shum, D. (2011). A quasi-experimental design trail exploring the effect of a partnership intervention on family and staff well-being in long-term dementia care. *Aging & Mental Health*, 15(8), 995–1007.

Bulechek, G., Butcher, H., Dochterman, J. & Wagner, C. (2013). *Nursing Interventions Classification (NIC)*. (6th edition). St Louis: Elsevier.

Hunter, S. (2012). *Miller's Nursing for Wellness in Older Adults*. Philadelphia: Wolters Kluwer/Lippincott Williams & Wilkins.

Kellett, U. (2007). Seizing possibilities for positive family caregiving in nursing homes. *Journal of Clinical Nursing*, 16, 1479–87.

King, A. (2001). *The Primary Health Care Strategy,* Retrieved from www.http://www.health.govt.nz

Maas, M., Buckwalter, K., Swanson, E., Specht, J., Tripp-Reimer, T. & Hardy, M. (1994). The caring partnership: Staff and families of persons institutionalised with Alzheimer's disease. *The American Journal of Alzheimer's Care and Related Disorders & Research, November/December 1994*, 21–9.

Maas, M., Reed, D., Park, M., Specht, J., Schutte, D., Kelley, L., ... Buckwalter, K. (2004). Outcomes of family involvement in care: Intervention for caregivers of individuals with dementia. *Nursing Research*, 53(2), 76–86.

Ministry of Social Development New Zealand. (2013). *A Guide for Carers*, Retrieved from http://www.msd.govt.nz/

Moyle, W. (2010). Is quality of life being compromised in people with dementia in long-term care? *International Journal of Older People Nursing*, 5(3), 245–52.

Moyle, W., Edwards, H. & Clinton, M. (2002). Living with loss: Dementia and the family caregiver. *Australian Journal of Advanced Nursing*, 19(3), 25–31.

Moyle, W., Murfield, J., Griffiths, S. & Venturato, L. (2011). Care staff attitudes and experiences of working with older people with dementia. *Australasian Journal on Ageing*, 30(4), 186–90.

New Zealand Department of Labour. (2011). *Labour Market Characteristics of Unpaid Carers*. Wellington.

Nolan, M., Bauer, M. & Nay, R. (2009). Supporting family carers: Implementing a relational approach. In R. Nay & S. Garratt (Eds.), *Nursing Older People: Issues and Innovations* (pp. 136–52). Sydney: Elsevier.

Nolan, M., Davies, S., Brown, J., Keady, J. & Nolan, J. (2004). Beyond 'person-centred' care: A new vision for gerontological nursing. *Journal of Clinical Nursing: International Journal of Older People Nursing*, 13(3(a)), 45–53.

Nolan, M., Grant, G., Keady, J. & Lundh, U. (2003). New directions for partnerships: Relationship-centred care. In M. Nolan, U. Lundh, G. Grant & J. Keady (Eds.), *Partnerships in Family Care*. Maidenhead: Open University Press.

Rees, G. (2013). Caring for older people: Issues for consumers. In R. Nay, S. Garratt & D. Fetherstone (Eds.), *Older People: Issues and Innovations in Care*. Sydney: Elsevier.

Statistics New Zealand. (2006). *Disability and Informal Care in New Zealand in 2006*. Wellington.

Stockwell-Smith, G., Kellett, U. & Moyle, W. (2010). Why carers of frail older people are not using available respite services: An Australian study. *Journal of Clinical Nursing*, 19, 2057–64.

Tabloski, P. (2010). *Gerontological Nursing*. (2nd edition). New Jersey: Pearson.

9 Evidence-based nursing interventions: fostering quality of life

Wendy Moyle

Learning objectives

After reading this chapter you will be able to:

1 Define quality of life (QOL) and health-related quality of life (HRQoL).

2 Outline a nursing intervention that may foster QOL.

3 Outline some of the measurement scales of QOL that are available.

4 Describe levels of nursing evidence for nursing interventions.

5 Outline a nursing intervention that may be useful in your current nursing practice.

Introduction

This chapter focuses on evidence-based nursing interventions that aim to improve **quality of life** (QOL) of older people, with a particular focus on improving QOL of older people with dementia. The key to understanding whether a therapy or intervention is working is to consider objective measures such as response to treatment. Medical interventions focus on preventive, diagnostic, therapeutic or rehabilitative aims with outcomes being an improvement in health or alteration of disease. Nursing interventions in comparison tend to focus on improving quality of care. As an outcome of care and its impact on the essential elements of the health of the older person, nurses also need to consider subjective indicators such as QOL as a patient reported outcome. Indicators of QOL include emotional, physical and social functioning as well as home and family situation, satisfaction with life, health status, and chronic conditions such as pain, employment and access to health services (Fayers & Machin, 2007).

> **Quality of life**
> An individual's perception of their position in life in the context of the culture and value systems in which they live and in relation to their goals, expectations, standards and concerns.

What is quality of life?

Although indicators of QOL are reasonably clear, QOL is difficult to define. QOL means different things to different people. QOL is therefore a personal and variable concept and it needs to be considered within the area of application. For example it could relate to a drug trial that aims to improve the patient condition, or a broad social circumstance such as improving the environment through better housing. QOL can also be considered in a broad general sense. For example, a patient's QOL can be influenced by nursing care practice.

Where QOL measurement is being used as an indicator of treatment success on a particular disease, the term 'health related quality of life' (HRQoL) is frequently used. Like QOL, HRQoL is also a broad term but a number of factors are generally included in its definition. For example, HRQoL refers to 'general health, physical functioning, physical symptoms and toxicity, emotional functioning, cognitive functioning, role functioning, social well-being and functioning, sexual functioning and existential issues' (Fayers & Machin, 2007, p. 4).

Measurement of QOL is important as it helps us to understand the needs and desires of patients, and measurement of QOL can also help to improve nursing practice. QOL is measured using a measurement scale, which is a series of questions, ratings or items that are used to measure QOL outcomes for individual patients. There are a number of QOL measurement scales available, some being generic while others are disease specific measures. Examples of generic QOL measurement scales include: the Nottingham Health Profile (Hunt, McEwen & McKenna, 1985), which measures emotional, social and physical distress, and the Short Form 36 (SF-36) (Ware et al., 1993), which measures physical, social and emotional functioning. There are also disease specific measures such as the Hospital Anxiety and Depression Scale (Zigmond & Snaith, 1983), which is used to detect anxiety and depression. A good QOL measurement scale should be easy for patients or proxies, such as staff and family, to use and have the capacity to detect change in the patient's QOL.

Measurement of QOL can be challenging if a person has a cognitive impairment such as dementia. Moyle and Murfield (2013) found HRQoL difficult to measure because of the decline of memory and function in clients with dementia. When measuring HRQoL, therefore, they found that the domains that can be measured are usually behavioural competence, psychological well-being, objective environment and perceived HRQoL (Moyle & Murfield, 2013). The patient can rate their QOL. When a person's cognitive status no longer allows an evaluation, a proxy, such as a nurse or family member, may be asked to assess their HRQoL instead.

The Quality of Life of Alzheimer's Disease (QOL-AD) Scale (Logsdon et al., 2002) is a brief measure of HRQoL. Taking 5–15 minutes to complete, it is used by either the person living with dementia or their proxy. The questionnaire is based on literature reviews of QOL in older people. It has 13 items covering the areas of physical health, energy, mood, living situations, memory, family, marriage, friends, chores, fun, money, self and life as a whole. (A copy of the QOL-AD is available at end of the chapter.) The QOL-AD can be used with individuals with mild to moderate dementia, while the proxy version is used with persons with severe dementia (Moyle & Murfield, 2013).

Nurses can assist in improving patients' HRQoL through psychosocial or physiological nursing interventions. Psychosocial interventions use educational, behavioural and/or cognitive approaches to treat or prevent a condition (Forsman, Nordmyr & Wahlbeck, 2011). Physiological nursing interventions aim to maintain physiological status, for example through acid–base management. This chapter focuses only on psychosocial interventions.

Nursing interventions

Nursing interventions are actions undertaken by a nurse to improve patient outcomes. Nursing interventions are also known as 'any treatment, based upon clinical judgment and knowledge that a nurse performs to enhance client outcomes' (Joanna Briggs Institute, 2011a, p. 1). In a care situation, the nurse assesses and determines the problem that needs to be addressed. The nurse then formulates an appropriate intervention plan (as proposed in this book) taking into account the patient's strengths and capabilities. The intervention is then implemented and this is then followed by an evaluation of the intervention to determine if a further course of action is required.

In some countries a classification system of nursing interventions has been developed. Researchers in the US for example have developed the **Nursing Interventions Classification** (NIC), which is a comprehensive, research-based, standardised classification of interventions that nurses perform. The NIC

Nursing Interventions Classification
A comprehensive, research-based, standardised classification of interventions that nurses perform.

interventions include physiological and psychosocial interventions. There are 554 interventions listed in the NIC (6th edition), which are grouped into 30 classes and seven domains (Bulechek et al., 2013). The NIC has been adopted in the US for use in standards, care plans, competency evaluation, nursing information systems and nursing education programs. Although NIC is often discussed in other countries it has not to date been adopted in Australia and New Zealand. However, as many nursing curricula refer to textbooks from North America, it is important to understand the purpose of the classification system.

As previously introduced in Chapter 5 the main two sources of evidence for nursing interventions can be identified in Cochrane Reviews and reviews undertaken by the Joanna Briggs Institute (JBI). Both sources aim to present the best available evidence on nursing interventions. The reviews conducted by the Cochrane Collaboration are perceived to identify the strongest level of evidence because they limit the interventions reviewed to **randomised controlled trials** (RCTs), which are considered to be the gold standard of research design. Reviews undertaken by the JBI are more inclusive of both qualitative and quantitative approaches. The JBI in the past used a rating scale of 'A to D' to rate effectiveness of nursing interventions but has recently changed the scale to 'A or B' for levels of evidence. A rating scale of 'A' is a strong recommendation for the nursing intervention while a rating of 'B' is a weak recommendation. Previous JBI reviews continue to use the 'A to D' rating scale. A rating scale of evidence often referred to in nursing literature is Melnyk and Fineout-Overholt's (2011) Level of Evidence of Interventions Rating Scale (see Table 9.1).

> **Randomised controlled trials** Used to test the efficacy and effectiveness of interventions and involve participants being allocated at random to receive several interventions, including a comparison or control.

TABLE 9.1 *Level of Evidence of Interventions Rating Scale*

Level 1 – Systematic review and meta-analysis of randomised controlled trials; clinical guidelines based on systematic reviews or meta-analyses
Level 2 – One or more randomised controlled trials
Level 3 – Controlled trial (no randomisation)
Level 4 – Case-control or cohort study
Level 5 – Systematic review of descriptive & qualitative studies
Level 6 – Single descriptive or qualitative study
Level 7 – Expert opinion

Source: Melnyk & Fineout-Overholt, 2011

The following sections of this chapter review several popular and evidence-based nursing interventions that can be used by nursing professionals with older adults. These reviews focus on chronic pain, management of older people in emergency departments and management of older people living with dementia. The reviews indicate the level of evidence for each of the reviews.

Nursing interventions for adult patients experiencing chronic pain

Chronic pain in older people represents the third most frequently identified health problem (Joanna Briggs Institute, 2011a, p. 1). Chronic pain is multifactorial and therefore requires nursing interventions that focus on psychological, physical and pharmacological factors. See also Chapter 13 which describes chronic pain management in relation to palliative care. A JBI (2011a) systematic review considered the effectiveness of non-pharmacological nursing interventions for chronic pain using the 'A to D' rating scale. This review included eight studies of which seven were RCTs and one was a quasi-randomised controlled trial. The JBI systematic review recommended the following as being of 'grade B' effectiveness, indicating moderate support that warrants consideration of application for chronic pain in older adults:

Cognitive behavioural therapy An individualised approach that helps the individual to learn or relearn healthier skills and habits and to reduce negative thoughts.

Psycho-education Education to help with the psychological stress of a condition such as pain.

Snoezelen A multi-sensorial stimulation of the primary senses, i.e. hearing, touch, taste, smell and sight, through stimulants such as essential oils and music.

Magnetic field therapy Involves the placing of magnetic devices on or near the body to relieve pain.

Guided imagery A program of directed thoughts and suggestions that guide a person towards a relaxed state.

- Listening to music is an effective short-term nursing intervention for older people suffering from osteoarthritis, articular pain, depression and disability.
- **Cognitive behavioural therapy** was also recommended as an intervention that may help to reduce non-malignant chronic pain and **psycho-education** may also reduce the severity of osteoarticular pain.
- Alternative complementary interventions such as **Snoezelen**, **magnetic field therapy** and **guided imagery** were also recommended as being useful for reducing chronic pain.
- Exercise programs may also be effective at improving physical function and therefore improving chronic pain in older patients.

Age-friendly nursing interventions in the management of older people in emergency departments

Older people are high users of emergency departments (EDs). However, such busy environments are not well designed for older people and as a result their condition may deteriorate as a result of their stay (Joanna Briggs Institute, 2011b). A JBI systematic review identified 16 papers – two research studies, seven expert opinion papers and seven policy papers – in the area of management of older people in EDs. Only one of the papers identified was a prospective RCT and one was a quasi-experimental design. The JBI systematic review made the following recommendations indicated as 'grade B' – moderate support that warrants consideration of application:

- Provide separate and quiet areas in the ED department for older people and provide equipment that is age friendly (e.g. large faced clocks) and treatment and care that respects the dignity and privacy of older people.
- Provision of age friendly care and assessment that incorporates the family carer and is openly communicated and streamlined.
- Awareness and incorporation of assessment and treatment that is age appropriate; that is, regular mobilising of the older person to the toilet, decubitus ulcer risk assessment, hydration and skin moisturisers.

The older person in the emergency department

Case scenario 9.1

Jenny, a single woman aged 88 years, is in hospital following a fall at home. A neighbour found Jenny lying on the floor of her bedroom and she was brought into a busy emergency department (ED) ward in an agitated state with an elevated temperature. She was assessed as having an infected leg wound. It was decided that she would require treatment in hospital. While waiting for a geriatric consultation Jenny was taken to a quiet area within the ED ward especially designed for older people.

While in the ED a member of the aged care emergency team assessed Jenny and identified that she was confused and agitated. A cognitive assessment indicated that she was disoriented and had short-term memory loss suggesting a delirium, possibly as a result of her infection. The aged care team prompted Jenny to eat and drink during her stay and provided cues such as a clock, television and books to orientate her to time and place. The team called Jenny's family and general practitioner and found there had been a gradual decline in her physical functioning over the last six months as Jenny had become frail. Following the geriatric consultation Jenny was admitted to a geriatric assessment ward.

The above case scenario indicates that there is early recognition of Jenny's physical and cognitive status. Her condition is treated quickly and the team prevent any additional complications while waiting in the ED ward through prompting her to eat and drink and providing orientation cues.

Reflective questions

Reflect on the case scenario and address the following questions:

› What prompted the ED team to assess Jenny in an ED ward designed for older people?

› What might have occurred if the ED team had not assessed Jenny's mental and cognitive status?

Reflective activity

Think about situations where you have seen older people being brought into an ED or a ward following a fall at home.

● What assessments were undertaken and what orientation processes were put into place?

● What aspects, if any, of the JBI recommendations were followed?

● What other JBI recommendations do you think could have been followed?

Nursing interventions in the management of older people with dementia

Dementia is a syndrome of cognitive deficits that involves both memory impairments and a disturbance in at least one other area of cognition, such as comprehension or production of speech (aphasia); certain motor movements (apraxia); interpretation of sensations and recognition of things (agnosia); or the management of cognitive processes (executive function). Nurses have a key role in the assessment and management of older people with dementia. The following sections outline recent evidence for several popular nursing interventions.

Aromatherapy for dementia

Four studies were included in a Cochrane Collaboration Review of aromatherapy for dementia (Holt et al., 2003). Only one study (Ballard et al., 2002) identified a statistically significant treatment effect in reducing agitation and neuropsychiatric symptoms; however, several methodological issues were reported in relation to this study. The review suggested further large scale RCT designed research was required. A recent single, blinded RCT of 67 people with a diagnosis of dementia and a history of agitated behaviour from three long-term care facilities were randomised into three groups: group one was a combination group receiving aromatherapy (3% lavender oil) and hand massage; group two received aromatherapy (3% lavender oil spray); and group 3 was the control group receiving water spray each twice daily for six weeks (Fu, Moyle & Cooke, 2013). The authors of this study found that, despite a downward trend in agitation, the aromatherapy intervention did not significantly reduce disruptive behaviour. The current evidence is therefore not strong for aromatherapy use. However, Fu, Moyle and Cooke (2013) also recommended that further large scale RCT studies were required.

Psychosocial interventions for reducing anti-psychotic medication in care home residents

Anti-psychotic medication is regularly prescribed in long-term care to manage **behavioural and psychological symptoms of dementia** (BPSD). Such treatment has a number of adverse effects such as falls (related to the sedative effects), constipation and incontinence. A Cochrane Collaboration Systematic Review (Richter et al., 2012) identified four cluster RCTs that investigated complex nursing interventions comprising educational approaches, all with the aim to reduce anti-psychotic medication use. Three of the selected studies offered education and training to the nursing staff and the fourth study offered an intervention composed of multidisciplinary team meetings. The methodological quality of the studies was moderate. The four studies all reported a decrease in anti-psychotic drug treatment use and suggested the positive evidence for education interventions targeting care professionals.

> **Anti-psychotic medication**
> A class of medication that is used to treat psychosis, as well as mental and emotional conditions.
>
> **Behavioural and psychological symptoms of dementia**
> Distressing and non-cognitive symptoms of dementia such as agitation and aggression.

Massage and touch for dementia

Hansen and colleagues (2006) carried out a Cochrane Collaboration Review on massage and touch. Their review indicated that massage and touch might be offered to people with dementia as an intervention to reduce agitation and incite comfort. These two interventions are often considered as being able to reduce depression, anxiety and aggression (Cohen-Mansfield, 2001). Touch is also considered to have an immediate calming influence as a result of oxytocin stimulus (Lund et al., 2002). Two studies met the Hansen, Jørgensen & Ørtenblad (2006) methodological criteria. Although small in number the studies indicated evidence for hand massage as a means to bring about short-term reduction in agitated behaviour, and touch and verbal encouragement to help people with dementia maintain eating patterns .

A recent RCT by Moyle et al. (2013a) sought to compare the effect of foot massage (10 minute massage five times a week for three weeks) with quiet presence (a control group where the only interaction was the carer sitting with the resident). The study findings indicated an increase in agitation in both the intervention and control group. There was also a trend towards a positive change in alertness in the foot massage group (indicating reduced alertness) and a negative change for residents in the quiet presence group (indicating increased alertness). The researchers highlighted the contribution the unfamiliar therapists may have made to an increase in agitation and recommended further research. This research supports the need to focus on interventions targeted at individual needs and the importance of nursing professionals being familiar to patients and being able to identify their needs.

The following two nursing interventions are often found in use in long-term care. However, neither have received either Cochrane Collaboration or JBI review possibly because the research available to date is not extensive and in the case of the social robots the technology is new and therefore there is still limited understanding of their benefits.

Nursing interventions using pet therapy

Scientific evidence for pets as therapy was first outlined in the 1970s. Katcher (1977) found that pets lowered blood pressure and Friedmann et al. (1980) found that pets also positively influenced survival rates in pet owners. Since this time there has been an increase in the number of published pet therapy studies, however most of the studies are small in sample size and there is a lack of replication or longitudinal studies. A recent review of the literature explored whether residents living in long-term care who engaged in dog therapy had improved QOL outcomes (Cipriani et al., 2013). Nineteen studies met the authors' inclusion criteria and these were reviewed using the

McMaster's Critical Review Form – Quantitative Studies. Of the 19 studies three were randomised controlled trials, 11 cohort studies, four pre-post studies and one single case design. Fourteen of the studies reported having participants with Alzheimer's disease. Twelve reported statistically significant improved QOL outcomes for residents, although several limitations were reported in relation to study design and sample size. Cipriani et al. (2013) recommended further research that included larger sample sizes and single subject designs, as well as RCT design and validated instruments and outcome measures.

Nursing interventions using companion robots

Robotic animals have in recent years been introduced into long-term care as companions for persons with cognitive impairment. The early work of Libin and Cohen-Mansfield (2004) identified the advantages of robotic animals as their highly lifelike appearance and behaviour as well as their ability to model emotional states of older people. Such robots also provide the opportunity for comfort through stroking, cuddling and communication. Although some studies (Kramer, Friedmann & Bernstein, 2009; Tamura et al., 2004; Wada & Shibata, 2007) have reported improvements in QOL, relationships and loneliness in older people using robotic animals, to date these findings have been confined by methodological limitations such as small sample sizes and no control groups. A small scale pilot project evaluating the effect of a companion robot called PARO on mood and QOL of people with dementia aimed to overcome these methodological concerns while supporting evidence for further studies (Moyle et al., 2013b).

PARO is a therapeutic companion robot developed by Dr Takanori Shibata from Japan. PARO has the appearance of a baby harp seal and its tactile sensors, including eye opening in response to petting, encourage a very lifelike response. A study by Moyle et al. (2013b) using both an intervention (PARO) and control (reading) group for 45 minutes, three afternoons per week, for five weeks identified improvements in QOL (QOL-AD, 0.6 – 1.3) and pleasure (0.7) in the PARO group compared to the control group. There were also reductions in anxiety in the PARO group compared to the control group. Although the findings are positive the authors also indicated the need for a larger study.

mpanion robots and the person with dementia

Case scenario 9.2

Joan is 80 years old. She has lived in the nursing home for six months following a diagnosis of dementia and family concerns that she was not attending to her activities of daily living. Joan tended to isolate herself within the nursing home and appeared withdrawn and sad. Staff were keen to involve Joan in an activity that might bring joy and quality back into her life. Joan's family agreed for her to participate in a PARO study. At the first research group session Joan sat quietly waiting for her turn to hold PARO. When given PARO her face lit up, she smiled, spoke to PARO and hugged PARO closely when PARO responded positively to her stroking. Joan appeared excited by the intervention and she spoke to staff and her family about the PARO seal. Joan enjoyed each PARO session and by the third week she decided to take an even more active role as a group facilitator, taking PARO to each participant, showing participants what PARO could do, while talking softly to PARO.

PARO offered Joan the opportunity for comfort, companionship and also the opportunity to facilitate her interaction within the group. Joan had been a teacher in her past life and PARO had triggered her education capability and strength and offered her to the opportunity to do what she knew best – to help others through her teaching.

Reflective questions

Read and reflect on this case scenario and address the following questions:

> Why do you think Joan might have enjoyed the PARO robot?

> What needs might the PARO robot have offered to Joan that she was not having fulfilled?

> What were Joan's strengths and how did the activity build on those strengths?

Reflective activity

Think of a time when you or nursing staff have identified a patient as appearing sad and non-communicative.

● Were nursing interventions put into place to help this patient?
● If so, did they focus on the individual's strengths and capabilities?
● Did they help the patient?
● If no nursing interventions were put into place, why not?
● What do you think might have helped the patient?
● How might you have actioned such an intervention?

Summary

- Quality of life is difficult to define as it is an individual response.
- Health related quality of life is an important indicator of quality of life.

- There are numerous psychosocial nursing interventions that can be used by the nursing profession to improve a patient's quality of life. However, when choosing, a focus on the individual needs/condition will help to achieve a positive patient outcome.
- To improve quality of life we must deliver nursing interventions that have strong evidence for their use.
- The Cochrane Collaboration and JBI websites can help us to identify nursing interventions with strong evidence for their use.

Conclusion

This chapter examined the topic of quality of life and health related quality of life. The chapter outlined ways to assist patients to improve these areas. Further, the chapter discussed nursing interventions and the importance of understanding the levels of evidence available for the myriad of nursing interventions available. The chapter finished with an outline of potential nursing interventions that may be suitable for older people in the situations of chronic pain, management in emergency departments and dementia. Nursing practices that are grounded in research and based on the best available evidence will result in positive outcomes for older people.

Further reading

You may also like to refer to the Hartford Institute for Geriatric Nursing for nursing interventions related to specific geriatric conditions at: http://consult-gerirn.org/about

References

Ballard, C., O'Brien, J., Reichelt, K. & Perry, E. (2002). Aromatherapy as a safe and effective treatment for the management of agitation in severe dementia: The results of a double-blind, placebo-controlled trial with Melissa. *Journal of Clinical Psychiatry*, 63(7), 553–8.

Bulechek, G., Butcher, H., Dochterman, J. & Wagner, C. (Eds.). (2013). *Nursing Interventions Classification (NIC)*. (6th edition). St. Louis: Elsevier.

Cipriani, J., Cooper, M., DiGiovanni, N., Litchkofski, A., Nichols, A. & Ramsey, A. (2013). Dog-assisted therapy for residents of long-term care facilities: An evidence-based review with implications for occupational therapy. *Occupational Therapy in Geriatrics*, 31(3), 214–40.

Cohen-Mansfield, J. (2001). Nonpharmacological interventions for inappropriate behaviors in dementia. *American Journal of Geriatric Psychiatry*, 9(4), 361–81.

Fayers, P. & Machin, D. (2007). *Quality of Life. The Assessment, Analysis and Interpretation of Patient Reported Outcomes*. New Jersey: Wiley.

Forsman, A., Nordmyr, J. & Wahlbeck, K. (2011). Psychosocial interventions for the promotion of mental health and the prevention of depression among older adults. *Health Promotion International*, 26, i85–i107.

Friedmann, E., Katcher, A., Lynch, J. & Thomas, S. (1980). Animal companions and one-year survival of patients after discharge from a coronary care unit. *Public Health Report*, 95(4), 307–12.

Fu, C., Moyle, W. & Cooke, M. (2013). A randomised controlled trial of the use of aromatherapy and hand massage to reduce disruptive behaviour in people with dementia. *BMC Complementary and Alternative Medicine*, 13, 165.

Hansen, N., Jørgensen, T. & Ørtenblad, L. (2006). Massage and touch for dementia. *Cochrane Database of Systematic Reviews*. doi: 10.1002/14651858.CD004989.pub2

Holt, F., Birks, T., Thorgrimsen, L., Spector, A., Wiles, A. & Orrell, M. (2003). Aromatherapy for dementia. *Cochrane Database of Systematic Reviews*. doi: 10.1002/14651858.CD003150

Hunt, S., McEwen, J. & McKenna, S. (1985). Measuring health status: A new tool for clinicians and epidemiologists. *Journal Royal College of General Practitioners*, 35(273), 185–8.

Joanna Briggs Institute. (2011a). *Nursing intervention for adult patients experiencing chronic pain. Best Practice: Evidence-based Information Sheets for Health Professionals*. 15(10), 1–4

Joanna Briggs Institute. (2011b). *Age-friendly nursing interventions in the management of older people in emergency departments. Best Practice: Evidence-based Information Sheets for Health Professionals*. 15(16): 1–4

Katcher, A. (1977). Physiologic and behavioural responses to companion animals. *Pyschosomatic Medicine*, 39(3), 188–92.

Kramer, S., Friedmann, E. & Bernstein, P. (2009). Comparison of the effect of human interaction, animal-assisted therapy, and AI-BO assisted therapy on long-term care residents with dementia. *Anthrozoos*, 22, 43–57.

Libin, A. & Cohen-Mansfield, J. (2004). Therapeutic robocat for nursing home residents with dementia: Preliminary inquiry. *American Journal of Alzheimer's Disease and Other Dementias*, 19, 111–16.

Logsdon, R., Gibbons, L., McCurry, S. & Teri, L. (2002). Assessing quality of life in older persons with cognitive impairment. *Psychosomatic Medicine*, 64(3), 510–19.

Lund, I., Long-Chuan, Y., Uvnas-Moberg, K., Wang, J., Yu, C., Kurosawa, M., … Lundeberg, T. (2002). Repeated massage-like stimulation induces long-term effects on nociception: Contribution of oxytocinergic mechanisms. *European Journal of Neuroscience*, 16(2), 330–8.

Melnyk, B. & Fineout-Overholt, E. (2011). *Evidence-based Practice in Nursing and Healthcare: A Guide to Best Practice*. Philadelphia: Lippincott, Williams & Wilkins.

Moyle, W., Cooke, M., Beattie, E., Shum, D., O'Dwyer, S. & Barrett, S. (2013a). Foot massage versus quiet presence on agitation and mood in people with dementia: A randomized controlled trial. *International Journal of Nursing Studies*. doi: 10.1016/j.ijnurstu.2013.10.019

Moyle, W., Cooke, M., Beattie, E., Jones, C., Klein, B., Cook, G. & Gray, C. (2013b). Exploring the effect of companion robots on emotional expression in older people with dementia: A pilot RCT. *Journal of Gerontological Nursing*, 39 (5), 46–53. doi: 10.3928/00989134–20130313–03

Moyle, W. & Murfield, J. (2013). Health-related quality of life in older people with severe dementia: Challenges for measurement and management. *Expert Review of Pharmacoeconomics and Outcome Research*, 13(1), 109–22.

Richter, T., Meyer, G., Möhler, R. & Köpke, S. (2012). Psychosocial interventions for reducing antipsychotic medication in care home residents. *Cochrane Database of Systematic Reviews*. doi: 10.1002/14651858.CD008634.pub2

Tamura, T., Yonemitsu, S., Itoh, A., Oikawa, D., Kawakami, A., Higashi, Y., ... Nakajima, K. (2004). Is an entertainment robot useful in the care of elderly people with severe dementia? *Journals of Gerontology Series A, Biological Sciences and Medical Sciences*, 59, 83–5.

Wada, K. & Shibata, T. (2007). Living with seal robots. Its sociopsychological and physiological influences on the elderly at a care house. *IEEE Transactions on Robotics*, 23, 972–80.

Ware, J. Jr, Snow, K., Kosinski, M. & Gandek, B. (1993) *SF-36 Health Survey Manual and Interpretation Guide*. Boston: New England Medical Centre.

Zigmond, A. & Snaith, R. (1983). The Hospital Anxiety and Depression Scale. *Acta Psychiatrica Scandinavica*, 67: 361–70.

Appendix: Quality of Life Questionnaire

QOL-AD[1]

Instructions: Interviewer administers according to standard instructions. Circle participant responses.

1. Physical health	Poor	Fair	Good	Excellent
2. Energy	Poor	Fair	Good	Excellent
3. Mood	Poor	Fair	Good	Excellent
4. Living situation	Poor	Fair	Good	Excellent
5. Memory	Poor	Fair	Good	Excellent
6. Family	Poor	Fair	Good	Excellent
7. Marriage	Poor	Fair	Good	Excellent
8. Friends	Poor	Fair	Good	Excellent
9. Self as a whole	Poor	Fair	Good	Excellent
10. Ability to do chores around the house	Poor	Fair	Good	Excellent
11. Ability to do things for fun	Poor	Fair	Good	Excellent
12. Money	Poor	Fair	Good	Excellent
13. Life as a whole	Poor	Fair	Good	Excellent

Source: Logsdon et al., 2002, pp. 510–19

[1] The QOL-AD is administered to individuals with dementia in interview format. For specific interview instructions, contact the author of the scale at logsdon@uw.edu.

3

End of life care

10 Palliative care in Australia and New Zealand

Deborah Parker

Learning objectives

After reading this chapter you will be able to:

1   Have an understanding of the historical and sociological development of palliative care in Australia and New Zealand.

2   Be aware of where older people die and the most common causes of death.

3   Describe the palliative care models for older adults in both community care and residential aged care.

4   Understand how to apply a strengths-based approach to palliative aged care for older people.

Introduction

This chapter focuses on palliative care for older people. Understanding the development of palliative care from a historical and sociological perspective provides a background to current services available to older people in Australia and New Zealand. Australia is one of the leading countries in the development of evidence-based guidelines for palliative care for older people and these are impacting on the way in which services are being developed and delivered.

Palliative care: definitions

The terms **hospice** and **palliative care** are sometimes used interchangeably. 'Hospice' can refer to a physical building where palliative care is provided, a philosophy of care or both. In Australia the term 'palliative care' describes the philosophy of care and 'hospices' or 'in-patient palliative care units' are the physical buildings. In New Zealand 'hospice' refers both to a physical building and a philosophy (Broad et al., 2013; Connolly et al., 2013). 'Hospice' was also traditionally linked to a cancer model of care (Maddocks, 1990). The most recent World Health Organization

Hospice
Physical building where care is provided (Australia); physical building and philosophy (New Zealand).

Palliative care
A philosophy of care.

definition of palliative care reflects the shift from palliative care being solely aligned with care of those with cancer to individuals with a life-threatening illness:

> Palliative care is an approach that improves the quality of life of patients and their families facing the problem associated with life-threatening illness, through the prevention and relief of suffering by means of early identification and impeccable assessment and treatment of pain and other problems, physical, psychosocial and spiritual. (World Health Organization, 2014)

Development of palliative care in Australia and New Zealand

The development of Australian and New Zealand palliative care services followed the emergence of the modern hospice movement in the UK, often highlighted by the establishment by Cicely Saunders of St Christopher's Hospice in London in 1967. The modern hospice philosophy and ideals emerged as a reformist approach to care, fuelled by the perceived inadequacy of the hospital system to provide humane care for the dying (Hunt & Maddocks, 1997; Mor, 1987; Seale, 1998). Prior to the opening of St Christopher's Hospice, religious organisations had been providing care for the dying, but these forerunner hospices had minimal skilled nursing and medical involvement. They did not achieve the status of those in the new movement, where holistic patient care was underpinned by research and education (Addington-Hall & Higginson, 2001; Hunt & Maddocks, 1997).

These reformist ideals of the new hospice movement appealed to the consumer public and resulted, in the UK, in rapid development and expansion of independent and voluntary hospices funded by charitable donations and operating outside of mainstream health care (McNamara, 1997). By the 1980s it became obvious that, for financial viability, integration with mainstream health care would be required. Today integration of hospice services with the UK National Health Service means less autonomy and more external scrutiny for their new service initiatives, which are now required to be based on needs assessment of the community, and not driven by interest groups (Clarke, 1993).

Australia's hospice development was, from the beginning, more aligned to mainstream health services. This was partly the result of a much smaller population than in the UK, restricting the emergence of the charitable and independent hospice sector. Prior to the 1980s religious orders had provided care for the terminally ill. The Order of the Little Company of Mary opened the Lewisham Hospital in Sydney in 1890 and Calvary Hospital in Adelaide in 1900. Further expansion occurred in 1938 with the opening in Melbourne of Caritas Christi Hospice, run by the Sisters of Charity. Twenty dedicated hospice beds were opened in the Mount Olivet Hospital in Brisbane and in 1964 the Little Company of Mary opened a 15 bed unit in Adelaide, the Mary Potter Wing of Calvary Hospital (Parker, 1997).

Hospice care development around the world led professionals, governments and academics to become more interested in promoting palliative care as a model of care. Needs analysis studies resulted in the establishment of palliative care programs in Western Australia and South Australia. A feature of development post-1980 was the establishment of state and national associations and an expansion of services through government funding with the development of accreditation guidelines (Harris & Finlay-Jones, 1987).

However, palliative services were not equally developed or accessible across Australia. As part of the 1988–89 federal budget, $37.8 million was allocated under the Medicare incentive packages (MIP) to identify and forward cost-effective programs for community palliative care support. Initially for five years, MIP was extended in 1993 for another five years and palliative care services were given further support by the Australian government with the establishment of the Palliative Care Program (Calder, 1998). As a result, palliative care service expansion across Australia has been rapid. In 1990, 122 hospice and palliative care services were listed in a national directory and in 2014 there are 227 supported by an extension network of primary care services.

This rapid expansion was supported by a National Palliative Care Strategy in 2002 and recently updated in 2010 (Commonwealth of Australia, 2010). This national strategy provided the basis for consolidation and funding national initiatives to improve research capacity, workforce education, improvements in quality care, affordable and available key medications for symptom control, and access to evidence to inform practice and policy. In New Zealand, the development of the Resource and Capability Framework for Integrated Palliative Care Services in New Zealand (2012) was aligned with the development work that had been undertaken in Australia.

Where do older people die and what do they die from?

In Australia during 2012, 147 098 people died with just over half (74 794) being male and 72 304 female. Most people who die are over the age of 65 years, the median age of death being 78.6 years for males and 84.6 years for females (Australian Bureau of Statistics, 2013). Leading causes of death across all ages are heart and circulatory disease, cancer, end stage organ failure, and dementia. The leading causes of death for people aged 65 years and over in Australia are ischaemic heart disease, cerebrovascular disease, lung cancer, chronic obstructive pulmonary disease, other heart disease and dementia (Australian Institute of Health and Welfare, 2007).

For those aged 65 years and over the·likelihood of living with dementia doubles every five years. Dementia was the third leading cause of death in 2010 (accounting for 6% of all deaths) and the number of deaths due to dementia increased 2.4 times between 2001 and 2010 (from 3740 to 9003 deaths). Dementia was recorded as the underlying or an additional cause of 14 per cent of deaths in 2010 (Australian Institute of Health and Welfare, 2012). The trajectory of dying with dementia is one of loss of physical and mental function; however, unlike a cancer trajectory these losses may occur over many years.

While it is common to hear that most people want to die at home, the reality is that more Australians die in a hospital, palliative care unit or residential aged care facility (RACF). In Australia, 32 per cent of people aged 65 years and over die in RACFs, which is similar to other developed countries. For New Zealand this represents 38 per cent of deaths, in Canada 30 per cent, in the US 28 per cent and in England 16 per cent (Broad et al., 2013). For people living with dementia, care in the community is usually possible in the early stages but as the disease progresses, and functional and mental capacity decrease, care in an RACF is usually required (Australian Institute of Health and Welfare, 2006).

Palliative care models for older adults

Palliative care is delivered across multiple settings – acute hospitals, primary care, generalist community services, neonatal and paediatric services, specialist palliative care settings, and residential aged care. Specialist palliative care services can provide support across non-specialist palliative care settings; however the extent of this support is not uniform across Australia. There is a diversity of models of palliative care across the different states and territories. This reflects specific local service delivery practices, health care systems and the demographics of the population that require care (Australian Institute of Health and Welfare, 2013a). New Zealand has a similar issue with access to palliative care dependent upon existing services, geographical location and diagnosis rather than the patient's assessed need. In both Australia and New Zealand, access to palliative care services is more limited for some population groups – Aboriginal and Torres Strait Islanders, Maori, rural populations, older people living in residential aged care and those with chronic illness (Commonwealth of Australia, 2010; Ministry of Health, 2012).

Because of the complexity of service delivery and inequity in access, governments in both Australia and New Zealand have advocated a needs-based approach to palliative care. Those with complex needs, regardless of diagnosis, should have access to specialist palliative care; those with intermediate needs should have access to periodic single specialist palliative care involvement; and those with straightforward needs can be cared for by primary care services. This needs-based approach also recognises that people across their care continuum may move between the different levels of needs (Palliative Care Australia, 2003).

The beginning of this chapter introduced the WHO definition of palliative care. While this definition can be applied to any person with a life-threatening illness, there are three terms used in Australia when people refer to the delivery of palliative care for older people. These are a **palliative approach**, **specialist palliative care** and **end of life care** (Department of Health and Ageing, 2006).

Palliative approach
The goal is to improve the person's level of comfort and function, and address physical, psychological, spiritual and social needs.

Specialist palliative care
Involves referral to a specialised palliative care team or health practitioner.

End of life care
Care in the last days or week of life.

A palliative approach

When the person's condition is not amenable to cure and the symptoms of the disease require effective symptom management, a palliative approach is appropriate. Providing active treatment for the disease may also still be important and may be provided concurrently with a palliative approach. The goal of a palliative approach is to improve the person's level of comfort and function, and to address their physical, psychological, spiritual and social needs (Department of Health and Ageing, 2006).

Specialist palliative care

Specialist palliative care involves referral to a specialised palliative team or health care practitioner. The focus is on assessing and treating complex symptoms experienced by the person; and providing information and advice on complex issues (for example, ethical dilemmas, family issues, or psychological or existential distress) to the aged care team (Department of Health and Ageing, 2006).

End of life care

End of life care is appropriate when the person is in the final days or weeks of life and care decisions may need to be reviewed more frequently. Goals are more sharply focused on the resident's physical, emotional and spiritual comfort, and support for the family (Department of Health and Ageing, 2006).

Specific details for older adults in RACFs and those still living in the community are discussed in the next section. In both instances the three forms of palliative care just described are present.

Residential aged care

In Australia, RACFs provide 24 hour nursing care for older people who are unable to stay in their own homes. At 30 June 2013, there were 2718 aged care facilities providing residential care in Australia with 74.6 per cent of places being used for high level care. Religious and charitable organisations provided the majority of services. In 2012–13 permanent care was provided to 226 042 people (Commonwealth of Australia, 2013). At 30 June 2012, 70 per cent of residents were female and women outnumbered men in every age group over age 70 (Australian Institute of Health and Welfare, 2013b). Residents are classified as **high care** or **low care** based on their **Aged Care Funding Instrument appraisal** (ACFI). At the same time, 80 per cent of permanent residents (133 411 people) were classified as high care; the remaining 38 941 appraisals were for low care (Commonwealth of Australia, 2013). At the same time, about 52 per cent of permanent residents with an ACFI appraisal had dementia. Residents with dementia were more likely than those without dementia to require high care (87% versus 63%) (Australian Institute of Health and Welfare, 2012, 2013b).

Between 1 July 2011 and 30 June 2012, there were 117 559 separations from RACFs. Of these, 49 per cent were permanent residents. Among permanent residents, the major reason for separation was death (91% of separations), while 4 per cent returned to the

High care
People who require almost complete assistance with most daily living activities as well as accommodation, meals, laundry and room cleaning.

Low care
People who require accommodation, meals, laundry, room cleaning as well as help with personal care and possibly nursing care.

Aged Care Funding Instrument appraisal
Used for determining the level of care payments for residents in residential aged care facilities.

community and 2 per cent moved to another residential aged care service. For permanent residents who separated from RACF during 1 July 2011 to 30 June 2012, 37 per cent were in care for less than 1 year, 44 per cent for between 1 and 5 years, and 18 per cent for 5 years or more. Nearly two-thirds (64%) of separations from respite care (see Chapter 4) were for residents returning to the community, about 17 per cent to another care service, and 3 per cent due to death (Australian Institute of Health and Welfare, 2013b).

New Zealand has a two tier system of care – rest homes provide support for their residents but are not required to provide 24 hour care; private hospitals provide 24 hour nursing/medical care. Similar to Australia 6.1 per cent of residents' deaths occur in private hospitals or rest homes within one month of admission and a further 16.2 per cent within six months (Broad et al., 2013).

No one specific model of providing palliative care in RACFs exists in Australia or New Zealand. Medical care for residents is provided by the residents' general practitioner (GP) and specialists visit on a consultative basis. The GP may or may not have skills and experience in providing palliative care. In some instances, specialist palliative care services provide consultancy directly to RACFs. However, in most instances support is limited. In Australia, the release in 2006 of the *Guidelines for a Palliative Approach in Residential Aged Care* (Department of Health and Ageing, 2006) provided the opportunity to develop a new model of palliative care. This model – A comprehensive evidence-based palliative approach in residential aged care (Parker, 2010) successfully demonstrated improved outcomes for residents by providing care based on resident prognosis and need. In this model, residents are classified into one of three trajectories and these in turn are linked to key care processes to assist staff to assess, plan and manage the palliative care needs of the resident and family. To assist all RACFs to implement this model, the Australian government has supported the development of the Palliative Approach Toolkit (Palliative Approach Toolkit, 2013). Detailed discussion of this model of care will be provided in Chapter 12 which focuses on palliative care in RACFs.

Community care

Most older people in Australia live in the community – either in their own homes, including in retirement villages, or with friends or relatives. As discussed above a small percentage of people aged 65 years and over live in an RACF. In Australia in 2011, 30 per cent of people with dementia lived in

RACF, while 70 per cent lived in the community (Australian Institute of Health and Welfare, 2012).

Delivering a palliative approach to care for older people in the community may involve multiple agencies and health care professionals. A collaborative approach that is well coordinated will provide a seamless and efficient care delivery. To assist health professionals working in this setting the *Guidelines for a Palliative Approach for Aged Care in the Community Setting – Best Practice Guidelines for the Australian Context* (Australian Government Department of Health and Ageing, 2011) were developed. These guidelines provide a comprehensive guide to the physical, social, psychological and spiritual care of older people as well as specific care for older people with special needs or perspectives such as dementia or neurological disease.

Unlike the model of care developed for RACFs, to date no one specific model of providing palliative care for older people in the community exists. This is partly due to the complexity of funding within community care as well as the more heterogeneous population that requires care. Three models of providing care for older people in the community are described below. They may exist individually or in combination:

1 Specialist palliative care model.
2 Case management model.
3 Consumer directed care model.

Specialist palliative care services are available for any individual living in the community with a life limiting illness. While they are more likely to be accessed by people with a cancer diagnosis, older people with organ failure or chronic diseases may be able to access specialist palliative care services. An approximate prognosis of less than three or six months to live may be applied depending on the service or the level of services requested. Specialist palliative care services are available within an in-patient hospital unit or specifically designed hospice although this care is usually reserved for short and rapid periods of worsening health, and decreasing independence before death. Where the care needs of older people extend over longer periods the most appropriate roles for specialist palliative care providers may be as consultants to aged care service providers (Kite, Jones & Tookman, 1999).

The case management model of care (Chapter 4) is often used to provide care for older adults who are eligible for a Home Care Package (previously Community Aged Care Packages (CACP), Extended Aged Care at Home (EACH) and Extended Aged Care at Home Dementia (EACHD) Packages (see Chapter 4). The model involves a case manager or coordinator who provides a single point of contact and coordinates the team and services involved in the care and support of the older person and their family (Diwan, Shugarman & Fries, 2004). While any members of the care team can be the coordinators for those requiring palliative care, nurses may be the most suitable. In Australia in 2012, 1 382 668 people received care through a home care package enabling people to be supported in the community until death. In 2011, 6.1 per cent of separations from CACPs were due to death and 32 per cent from EACH and EACHD packages (Australian Institute of Health and Welfare, 2012). Unfortunately, no data linkage is available to estimate how many of these clients also received care from specialist palliative care services.

Consumer Directed Care (CDC) (Chapters 4 and 8) gives older people a greater say and more control over the design and delivery of community care services provided to them and their carers via home care packages. The packages are identified as CDC Packaged Care (for care recipients) and Consumer Directed Respite Care (CDRC) for carers. CDC Packaged Care and CDRC allow older people and their carers to make choices about the types of care services they access and the delivery of those services, including who will deliver the services and when. Expected outcomes of the programs for both care recipients and carers include a better quality of life due to increased independence and empowerment over the services they are receiving (Commonwealth of Australia, 2011). From 1 August 2013, all new Home Care Packages must be delivered on a CDC basis. All packages from July 2015 will be consumer directed (KPMG, 2012). The extent to which the introduction of CDC will impact on older people remaining at home until death is not yet known. However, home death rates should at a minimum equal those under the previous system.

In any of these models where care needs are greater than can be provided by community care then entry of the older person in an RACF will be needed. This is particularly the case for those with a diagnosis of dementia.

A strengths-based approach to palliative aged care

You will recall from Chapter 3 that we discussed in detail the strengths-based approach to nursing care and how it could be applied to the care of older people. Just to recap, the strengths approach focuses on the identification and use

Life limiting illness

An illness in which it is expected that death will be a direct consequence.

of an individual's strengths and resources to problem solve and effect change (Cox, 2001). The strengths-based approach is particularly useful for older people with a **life limiting illness** as it encourages people to take a lead in their own care. In Chapter 3, Table 3.1 identified techniques to assist a strengths-based approach into practice. Let's revisit these with reference to how they apply to an older person with a life limiting illness (Table 10.1).

TABLE 10.1 *Techniques to assist a strengths-based approach into practice for older people with a life limiting illness*

TENET	TECHNIQUES
Self-determination	Advance care planning to document values and wishes at the end of life including place of preferred death.
Empowerment	A core value of palliative care is ensuring appropriate care is delivered where the person wishes to be cared for. This does not assume that care is required within an inpatient facility or residential aged care setting.
Collaboration	Provide opportunities for patients and staff to work together to provide the care required where possible in the place of choice.
Reflection on change	Provide opportunity for staff to hear patients' stories and use opportunity to mutually identify areas for future development.
Community engagement	Encourage patients, staff and families to identify supports within the community that can support the person in end of life care.
Regeneration	Encourage shared time for discussion between the individual, family, friends and caregivers in order to achieve goals within the time frame remaining.

Using a strengths-based approach to palliative care

Case scenario 10.1

Beryl is an 85 year old woman living alone in her own home. Beryl has end stage heart failure, non-insulin dependent diabetes, osteoarthritis and cataracts. She has three daughters, one who lives in the same city, the other two live interstate (3 hours' flight away). Beryl is receiving a Home Care Package Level 3 (previously EACH package) which provides assistance with some activities of daily living, assistance with meal preparation and medication administration. This package is administered by a church-based non-government provider. Beryl chose this provider as it has links with her local parish church where she has been a member all of her life.

Beryl's general practitioner (GP), who has been involved in her care for

many years, has recently suggested to her that she should make sure her affairs are in order including ensuring her family understand her wishes. While the GP could not put an exact time frame on how long Beryl had to live, he did indicate a possible six to 12 month prognosis. Beryl is unsure about putting things in writing and wonders why her three daughters can't just do the right thing when the time comes.

Reflective questions

You are a registered nurse providing case management for Beryl on her home care package.

› Using the strengths-based approach, what are the steps that you would undertake to ensure that Beryl has her values and wishes respected by her family and health professionals involved in her care?

› What role does Beryl's family play in helping her make decisions or following through those that she might want?

› What role would a specialist palliative care service play in Beryl's care now or in the future?

› How would you ensure that the current Home Care Package that your agency administers is used to support Beryl in maintaining her quality of life?

Summary

- The development of palliative care in Australia and New Zealand and the main causes of mortality influence how and where a palliative approach is provided for older adults.
- A strengths-based approach to care aligns with the philosophy of palliative aged care and enhances older people's opportunity to participate in decision making.

Conclusion

This chapter examined the historical development of palliative care in Australia and New Zealand and how this has influenced current care provision for older people. The strengths-based approach to nursing care aligns with the definition and philosophy of palliative care. Incorporating this into the care of older people who are dying will assist in ensuring their values and wishes are respected.

Further reading

You may like to take a look at the following reading recommendation: Caresearch at http://www.caresearch.com.au

References

Addington-Hall, J. & Higginson, I. (2001). Introduction. In J. Higginson (Ed.), *Palliative Care for Non-cancer Patients*. Oxford: Oxford University Press.

Australian Bureau of Statistics. (2013). *2013 Deaths Australia*. Canberra.

Australian Government Department of Health and Ageing. (2011). *Guidelines for a Palliative Approach for Aged Care in the Community Setting – Best Practice Guidelines for the Australian Context*. Canberra.

Australian Institute of Health and Welfare. (2006). *Dementia in Australia: National Data Analysis and Development.* Canberra.

Australian Institute of Health and Welfare. (2007). *Older Australia at a Glance.* (4th edition). Canberra.

Australian Institute of Health and Welfare. (2012). *Aged Care Packages in the Community 2010–11: A Statistical Overview. Aged Care Statistics Series No. 37.* Canberra.

Australian Institute of Health and Welfare. (2013a). *Palliative Care Services in Australia.* Canberra.

Australian Institute of Health and Welfare. (2013b). *Residential Aged Care and Aged Care Packages in the Community 2011–12.* Canberra.

Broad, J., Gott, M., Kim, H., Byd, M., Chen, H. & Connolly, M. (2013). Where do people die? An international comparison of deaths occurring in hospital and residential aged care settings in 45 populations, using published and unpublished available statistics. *International Journal of Public Health,* 58(2), 257–67.

Calder, R. (1998). Dimensions of change in health care: Implications for palliative care. In J. Aranda (Ed.), *Palliative Care: Explorations and Challenges.* Sydney: MacLennon and Petty.

Clarke, D. (1993). *Whither the Hospices?* Buckingham: Open University Press.

Commonwealth of Australia. (2010). *Supporting Australians to Live Well at the End of Life – National Palliative Care Strategy.* Canberra.

Commonwealth of Australia. (2011). *Community Packaged Care Guidelines Incorporating: Community Aged Care packages, Extended Aged Care at Home packages and Extended Aged Care at Home Dementia packages.* Canberra.

Commonwealth of Australia. (2013). *Report on the Operation of the Aged Care Act 1997.* Canberra.

Connolly, M., Broad, J., Boyd, M., Kerse, N. & Gott, M. (2013). Residential aged care: The de facto hospice for New Zealand's older people. *Australasian Journal on Ageing.* doi: 10.1111/ajag.12010

Cox, A. (2001). BSW students favor strengths/empowerment based generalist practice. *Families in Society,* 82, 305–13.

Department of Health and Ageing. (2006). *Guidelines for a Palliative Approach in Residential Aged Care Facilities – NHMRC Endorsed Edition.* Canberra. Retrieved from http://www.nhmrc.gov.au/publications/synopses/ac12to14syn.htm

Diwan, S., Shugarman, L. & Fries, B. (2004). Problem identification and care plan responses in a home and community-based services program. *Journal of Applied Gerontology,* 23(3), 193–211.

Harris, R. & Finlay-Jones, L. (1987). Terminal care in Australia. *The Hospice Journal,* 3(1), 77–90.

Hunt, R. & Maddocks, I. (1997). Terminal care in South Australia: Historical aspects and equity issues. In J. Clark (Ed.), *New Themes in Palliative Care.* Milton Keynes: Open University Press.

Kite, S., Jones, K. & Tookman, A. (1999). Specialist palliative care and patients with noncancer diagnoses: The experience of a service. *Palliative Medicine*, 13(6), 477–84.

KPMG. (2012). *Evaluation of the Consumer-Directed Care Initiative: Final Report.* Canberra.

Maddocks, I. (1990). Changing concepts in palliative care. *Medical Journal of Australia*, 1152, 535–9.

McNamara, B. (1997). *Good enough death: An ethnography of hospice and palliative care.* [PhD]. Perth: University of Western Australia.

Ministry of Health. (2012). *Resource and capability framework for integrated adult palliative care services in New Zealand.* Wellington.

Mor, V. (1987). *Hospice Care Systems: Structure, Process, Costs and Outcome.* New York: Springer Publishing Company.

Palliative Approach Toolkit. (2013). *National Rollout of the Palliative Approach Toolkit.* Retrieved, from http://www.caresearch.com.au/PAToolkit

Palliative Care Australia. (2003). *Palliative Care Service Provision in Australia: A Planning Guide.* Canberra.

Parker, D. (1997). *The construction of identities for people dying in residential aged care facilities.* [Unpublished doctoral dissertation]. Adelaide: Flinders University.

Parker, D. (2010). Palliative Care in Residential Aged Care. *Progress in Palliative Care*, 18(6), 352–7.

Seale, C. (1998). *Constructing Death – The Sociology of Dying and Bereavement.* Cambridge: Cambridge University Press.

World Health Organization. (2014). WHO definition of palliative care. [Search for 'definition of palliative care']. Retrieved from http://www.who.int/cancer/palliative/definition/en/

11
Advance care planning for the frail older adult

Deborah Parker

Learning objectives

After reading this chapter you will be able to:

1   Have an understanding of advance care planning and advance care directives in Australia and New Zealand.

2   Understand how to apply a strengths-based approach to advance care planning.

3   Be aware of the issues of advance care planning for people who are unable to participate; for example, those with dementia.

Introduction

Advance care planning
A process whereby a person's values, beliefs and preferences are made known so that they can be used to guide decision making in circumstances where the person is no longer able to do so.

This chapter focuses on **advance care planning** (ACP). Firstly we will look at the history of advance care planning before specifically focusing on the current practice of advance care planning in Australia and New Zealand. Next we will explore how a strengths-based framework to advance care planning can be used in your everyday practice and finally we will identify specific issues in advance care planning for people who are unable to participate such as people with dementia.

History of advance care planning

ACP, while not a new phenomenon, has in the last decade received increased attention in Australia and New Zealand. Internationally, the beginnings of advance care planning were driven largely by the consumer health movement in the late 1960s. At this time there was a push towards the reduction in unnecessary invasive treatment when people were dying. The US was the leader in this movement and by the late 1970s most US states had legislation such as living wills, do-not-resuscitate orders or do-not-hospitalise orders. In 1991 the US Patient Self-Determination Act was passed, which was a federal law that allowed for the appointment of substitute decision makers and the withdrawal of life support (Street & Ottman, 2006). Other countries followed the US trend and in Australia, the first legislation supporting advance care planning occurred during the 1980s in Victoria, New South Wales, Queensland, the Northern Territory and Tasmania. This was followed in the 1990s by South Australia and lastly by the ACT (2006) and Western Australia (2008).

Advance care planning in Australia

ACP is a process whereby a person's values, beliefs and preferences are made known so that they can be used to guide decision making in circumstances where the person is no longer able to do so. An ACP discussion may result in the development of an **advance care directive** (ACD) and/or the appointment of a **substitute decision maker** (Australian Health Ministers' Advisory Council, 2011).

An ACD is a legal document that sets out instructions that consent to or refuse specified medical treatments. It is designed to be enacted when the person is no longer able to make informed decisions. You may have heard other terms for advance care directives like advance directives, advance health directives or living wills. An ACD must be completed and signed by an adult who is considered competent to make decisions. An ACD can record the person's wishes and appoint a substitute decision maker (SDM). A substitute decision is made on behalf of a person who lacks capacity. The decision should reflect that which the person who has lost capacity would have made. There are different ACDs depending on which state or territory you are in Australia (see Table 11.1) (Australian Health Ministers' Advisory Council, 2011).

Advance care directive A legal document that sets out instructions that consent to or refuse specified medical treatments. It is designed to be enacted when the person is no longer able to make informed decisions.

Substitute decision maker Someone who acts on behalf of a person who lacks capacity.

You will notice, looking at Table 11.1, that there is a range of terms that are used and it is important to make sure you are aware of the legislation that relates to the state or territory you are practising in. This inconsistency between Australian states and territories in regard to ACD is being addressed. In 2011 *A National Framework for Advance Care Directives* was developed and in time it is anticipated that as new laws are passed or existing laws updated greater consistency will occur (Australian Health Ministers' Advisory Council, 2011).

TABLE 11.1 *Statute laws for advance directives and substitute decision making in Australia*

	Legislation	Advance care directive	Substitute decision maker
ACT	Powers of Attorney Act 2006	Enduring Power of Attorney (health decisions)	Attorney (must be authorised for health decisions)
	Medical Treatment (Health Directions) Act 2006	Health Direction	Attorney
NSW	Guardianship Act 1987	Enduring Power of Guardianship (health, personal and residential decisions)	Enduring guardian
NT	Natural Death Act 1988	Direction (medical decisions only limited to terminal illness)	None
QLD	Powers of Attorney Act 1998	Enduring Power of Attorney (health) and Enduring Power of Attorney (personal)	Attorney (if authorised to make health decisions)
	Guardianship and Administration Act 2000	Advance Health Directive (health decisions)	Statutory health attorney
SA	Advance Care Directives Act 2013	Advance Care Directive (health, personal and residential decisions) (From 1 July 2014, the former Enduring Power of Guardianship, Medical Power of Attorney and Anticipatory Direction will be legally recognised as if it was an Advance Care Directive made under the Act, but applied according to the terms of the document)	Instructions, wishes and preferences and/or substitute decision maker
TAS	Guardianship and Administration Act 1995	Enduring Power of Guardianship (health, personal and residential decisions)	Enduring guardian
VIC	Guardianship and Administration Act 1986	Enduring Guardianship (health, personal and residential decisions)	Enduring guardian
	Medical Treatment Act 1988	Enduring Power of Attorney (Medical Treatment) and	Medical agent
		Refusal of Treatment Certificate	None
WA	Guardianship and Administration Act 1990; Acts Amendment (Consent to Medical Treatment) Act 2008	Enduring Power of Guardianship (health, personal and residential decisions) Advance Health Directive (health decisions)	Enduring guardian None

It is also important to note that, in the event that someone does not appoint a substitute decision maker or there is no legislation to cover that appointment, there is in each state a hierarchy of persons responsible who are able to consent to or refuse health care for a person with impaired decision making capacity. In Western Australia this hierarchy is listed in Figure 11.1. You will note that at the top of the hierarchy is the Advance Health Directive (AHD). If the person has made an AHD which covers the treatment decision required, no one else is authorised to make that decision, as the AHD takes precedence. This means even an enduring guardian (next on the list) cannot override these decisions (Government of Western Australia, 2010). As there are some differences across Australia you should consult the appropriate legislation. (More details are provided at the end of the chapter.)

AHD

- Decisions must be made in accordance with the AHD unless circumstances have changed or could not have been foreseen by the maker.

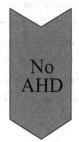

No AHD

- Enduring guardian with authority
- Guardian with authority
- Spouse or de facto partner
- Parent
- Sibling
- Primary unpaid carer
- Other person with close personal relationship

FIGURE 11.1   *Hierarchy in relation to treatment decisions in the enduring power of guardianship, Western Australia*

The extent to which ACP, including the uptake of ACDs, has been achieved in Australia is difficult to quantify. Currently, there is no mechanism by which people lodge at a state or federal level their advance care plan or ACD. National data on the existence of substitute decision makers is also not available. Various studies have estimated the use of advance care plan discussions between 1–29 per cent. In residential aged care the prevalence of AHDs in one study in New South Wales was 0.2 per cent (Nair et al., 2000). In a South Australian study 7 per cent of residents surveyed had appointed a medical power of attorney and 6 per cent had made an anticipatory directive (Brown et al., 2005). In a more recent national study, the rate of completion of advance health directives was 22 per cent (Parker, Hughes & Tuckett, 2011).

In Australia the Respecting Patient Choices (RPC) Program has been a major national initiative to improve ACP across all settings. It was adopted from a successful program in La Crosse in Wisconsin where during the mid-1980s a community wide approach to ACP using 'Respecting Patient Choices' was implemented. This program included patient education materials, training of local non-physician educators, who were available at all health care organisations, and common policies and practices of advance directive documents in all health care organisations. This study showed that 85 per cent of people who died during the study period had advance directives and 95 per cent of these were attached to the person's medical record (Hammes & Rooney, 1998). The authors compared this to a previous study within the area where 15 per cent of the individuals had a written ACD. The success of this program was the extent to which all health care providers in one geographical area participated.

The Australian RPC program has not had the same effectiveness as it has not been adopted within one geographical area by all health institutions. It has however demonstrated success for older people admitted to a public hospital. In a randomised control trial patients who were exposed to the RPC program and for whom ACP was discussed were more likely to have expressed their wishes in writing, appointed a proxy decision maker or both. Compared to a control group, who did not specifically have ACP discussed, family members of patients in the program were significantly less stressed, anxious and depressed (Detering et al., 2010).

Advance care planning in New Zealand

New Zealand has its own unique culture and legislation that differentiates ACP policy and practices from other countries. The Australian National Framework discussed above has not been completely adopted in New Zealand. Fundamental to all health approaches in New Zealand is the firm commitment to the cultural considerations of heritage, honouring Te Tiriti o Waitangi and recognising the cultural importance of involving the person's family or whanau. In New Zealand advance care plans are instructions made while a person is still capable and an advance care plan cannot be made for someone else. Similarly to Australia, the ACP process may result in the person choosing to write an advance care plan, and/or an advance directive, and/or to appoint an enduring power of attorney (EPA). While an advance care plan can be verbal, it is ideally completed on a form designed to capture the information that will be required to uphold a person's wishes. An advance care plan may itself be regarded as an advance directive and should be consistent with and considered in conjunction with any other advance directive that exists. It should be written in the knowledge that it could have legal authority. As yet in New Zealand there has been no legal test that a written advance care plan would constitute an advance directive for legal purposes (Ministry of Health New Zealand, 2011).

Advance directives are instructions on what medical care or treatment a person chooses. They may be oral or written. There are four legal criteria for an advance directive to be valid:

1   The person must be competent at the time of making the directive.
2   The decision they make to refuse treatment should have been made freely without pressure from anyone else.
3   At the time of making the advance directive, the intended refusal or consent to treatment should be applied in the situation where it will be used.
4   The existence and validity of the advance directive must be clearly established.

While there are no standard formats for advance directives, the New Zealand Medical Association has sample forms available at: http://nzma.org.nz/patients-guide/advance-directive (Ministry of Health New Zealand, 2011).

When should an advance care planning discussion occur?

ACP discussions can occur at any time. It is most likely that these will be raised when a person has been diagnosed with a life limiting illness. However in some instances older people may spontaneously bring up this topic with their family or general practitioner (GP). While more often people expect a health care professional to initiate discussions about ACP, as a nurse you should be prepared that anyone of any age who you are providing care for may want to discuss their wishes regarding treatment.

In particular the following circumstances are often triggers to begin discussing ACP:

- If a person or their family enquires about palliative care for a life limiting illness.
- If a person has been hospitalised recently for a severe progressive illness or condition, or has required repeated admissions for a serious condition.
- If a person says they want to forgo life sustaining treatment.
- If a person expresses a wish to die (Ministry of Health New Zealand, 2011).

For ACP to be successful the onus cannot be with one sector of the health system. ACP is a community wide issue and should be promoted in a similar manner to organ donation.

Advance care plans in residential aged care facilities

For individuals who require admission to a residential aged care facility (RACF), there are arguments for and against initiating the discussion of ACP on admission. The newly admitted resident and family may be stressed by the process of admission which is often precipitated by an acute event and following a period of hospitalisation. However, not raising issues of ACP on admission often leads to the next opportunity for such discussion occurring in a period of crisis or sudden event, and residents and families are stressed at this time as well. Two opportunities arise when ACP should be discussed in residential aged care. The first is on completion of the first care plan, which is usually part of a structured case conference within the first three months of admission. The second is when a person's condition deteriorates or goals of care need reviewing. In this instance the scheduling of a palliative care case conference can incorporate ACP (Parker et al., 2011; Shanley et al., 2009).

In 2009, the Respecting Patient Choices Program developed a specific advance care plan for use in RACFs. The plan has seven parts which include documentation of:

1 Existence of a medical power of attorney.
2 Current state of health.
3 Values and beliefs.
4 Future health situations.
5 Specific treatments (wanted and not wanted).
6 Goals for end of life care.

7 A final section where one of three boxes is selected. In summary these are:

   i   the option of refusing life prolonging treatment

   ii   to be transferred to hospital

   iii   for doctors and others the person has listed to make decisions for them.

The form has options for a competent person to sign or a declaration by the medical power of attorney as representative. A signature by the doctor and staff member is also required. An audit of the use of this new plan in 13 Victorian RACFs found that 49 per cent included the appointment of a medical power of attorney. Of the three options under request 73 per cent indicated the option of refusing life prolonging treatment, 12 per cent nominated the doctor to make medical decisions and 6 per cent wanted transfer to hospital for assessment and treatment (Silvester et al., 2013). It should be noted that this form is not an advance care directive covered by statute law but rather an advance care plan under common law.

To assist the uptake of ACP in any institutional setting requires a systematic approach including clear guidelines, polices, checklists and identification of responsibility for initiating and documenting the discussions (Shanley et al., 2009). Health professionals should be well prepared for these discussions, including allowing sufficient time, having enough knowledge about the person's clinical circumstances – including specific prognostic information – and being aware of the legal framework in which they are working (Australian Health Ministers' Advisory Council, 2011; Ministry of Health New Zealand, 2011).

A strengths-based framework for advance care planning

ACP is an ideal opportunity to work with older people to ensure wishes are respected. The ethical basis behind medical decision making is the principle of autonomy. In this context autonomy is defined as respect for the right of an individual to make their own decisions with regard to their own health and future. Reflecting back on the strengths-based approach to care that is featured in this book, we can see that ACP meets the tenets of the strengths approach to practice, in particular the focus on self-determination. Effective ACP encourages conversations about what is important for a person and helps a person achieve a sense of control as their illness progresses and death approaches.

It also engages others, including family and caregivers, to help them understand the person's wishes and to support them through the process. It also reassures the person that their wishes will be respected (Ministry of Health New Zealand, 2011). There is a range of ways to approach having an ACP discussion. The **Palliative Approach Toolkit** (University of Queensland, 2012), which will be discussed in detail in Chapter 12, has a step by step guide to conducting an ACP discussion (see below). While it is designed for nurses working in RACFs the principles are relevant regardless of setting.

> **Palliative Approach Toolkit**
> An evidence-based resource for providing a palliative approach in residential aged care facilities.

Steps to conducting an advance care planning discussion

Step 1 – Introduce ACP
Ask if the resident has thought about their choices of medical treatment in the future.

> 'How can we help you live well?' may be a less threatening reframe to commence discussions, allowing for a gradual lead into more sensitive questions.

Step 2 – Experience of end of life decision making

> Ask the resident if they have had any experience with a family member or friend who was faced with a decision about medical care near the end of life.
> If yes, ask them if the experience was positive or if they wished things could have been different and how.

Step 3 – Selecting a substitute decision maker

> Ask whom they would like to make decisions for them if they were unable to make their own choices known.
> If they have someone in mind, recommend that they discuss their wishes with their potential representative.
> Provide information on appointing a representative. See Table 11.1 for

information on state-based guidelines and legislation.

> A visit to the resident by a legal representative or counsel may be required. Ensure an appropriate level of privacy and provide assistance when needed.

Step 4 – Making decisions about future care

> Ask how they would like decisions to be made if they could no longer make those decisions.
> ACP discussions can encompass issues like:
> – beliefs and attitudes towards death and dying
> – active versus palliative treatments
> – resuscitation wishes
> – hospital admissions/ transfers
> – funeral wishes.

Step 5 – Goals and values

> Discuss with the resident what gives their life meaning. Possible responses might be specific beliefs, possessions, experiences, activities or relationships.

Step 6 – Religious, spiritual and cultural beliefs

> Ask who, or what, sustains them when they face serious challenges in life.

> Check if there is someone they would like to speak with to help them think about these issues.

> Be aware that cultural customs may differ with respect to patient autonomy, informed decision making, truth telling and control over the dying process.

Step 7 – Documenting ACP

Option 1 – The person may choose to complete an ACD using legislation in the state that is applicable including appointing a substitute decision maker.

Option 2 – The completion of an advance care plan.

Advance care planning for people unable to participate

A recent study by Alzheimer's Australia found that 69 per cent of care professionals felt that their organisation encouraged people with dementia to complete an advance care plan. However 20 per cent of family carers surveyed were dissatisfied with how health professionals adhered to the person's wishes and 31 per cent of care professionals experienced a situation where they did not feel they followed a person's wishes (Alzheimer's Australia, 2014). These findings indicate that there are still improvements in ensuring the care wishes of this vulnerable group are met and that there is still uncertainty among health professionals regarding ACP in this population.

For people living with early stage dementia there is opportunity to participate in ACP, complete a written advance directive and/or appoint a decision maker. A diagnosis of dementia does not automatically exclude people from these activities. In Australia, an adult has the capacity to make a decision when they can: understand the information being given; make a decision on the basis of the information given, after having weighed and fully appreciated the positive and negative consequences; and communicate that decision to another person (Alzheimer's Australia, 2005). A useful document from Capacity Australia (www.capacityaustralia.org.au) identifies that capacity is decision specific in recognising that a person's capacity may vary in different circumstances and at different times. They advocate the use of the ASKME Model of Supported Decision Making which fits well with our strengths-based approach to ACP.

This model is:

Assess strengths and deficits

Simplify the task

Know the person

Maximise the ability to understand

Enable participation.

Advance care planning – starting the conversation

Case scenario 11.1

You met Beryl in Chapter 10. Just to recap, she is an 85 year old woman living alone in her own home. Beryl has end stage heart failure, non-insulin dependent diabetes, osteoarthritis and cataracts. She has three daughters, one who lives in the same city, the other two live interstate (3 hours' flight away). Beryl is receiving a Home Care Package Level 3 (previously EACH package). Beryl's GP indicated that she had a possible six to 12 month prognosis.

Since you last met Beryl her daughters have become concerned about her cognitive ability. She seems to be more forgetful and when she phones to speak to them she tells them the same stories over and over. Sometimes she doesn't seem to know what the day or date is, however she is still pretty clear about what she does and doesn't want to do when it comes to her care and personal matters.

Reflective questions

You are the care coordinator and Beryl's daughter asks you about preparing an advance care plan.

〉 What should do in preparation for this discussion?

〉 Who should be involved in this discussion – other health professionals, family members, Beryl?

〉 How would you assess whether Beryl has the ability to participate in the discussion and complete an advance care plan?

〉 Who might help you with this decision?

Reflective activity

Reflect on an older person you know either personally or have cared for.

● How would you have approached having a conversation about ACP?

● What areas of the ACP did you find most difficult? Why?

● What sorts of questions do you think would be most difficult for you to ask an older person who you are caring for?

● Go back to the 'Steps to conducting an advance care planning discussion' box and see how this step by step process might help you with ACP discussions in the future.

Summary

- Advance care planning is supported in Australia and New Zealand by legislation.
- Advance care planning supports a strengths-based approach to care for older people.
- Special consideration is required for people who are unable to participate in advance care planning for example for those with dementia.

Conclusion

This chapter provided an overview of advance care planning in Australia and New Zealand. It is important to know the legislation that applies to your practice setting. Advance care planning is an opportunity for people to express their wishes so that these are respected in the event that they are no longer able to make decisions. Early advance care planning for older people is important.

Further reading

You may like to take a look at the following reading recommendations:

- Further information on ACP in Australia is available at: http://advance-careplanning.org.au/
- Further information on ACP in New Zealand is available at: http://www.advancecareplanning.org.nz/
- You may also like to refer to the Caresearch website: http://www.care-search.com.au

References

Alzheimer's Australia. (2005). *Legal Planning and Dementia*. Canberra.

Alzheimer's Australia. (2014). *End of Life Care for People with Dementia. Survey Report Executive Summary*. Canberra.

Australian Health Ministers' Advisory Council. (2011). *A National Framework for Advance Care Directives*. Canberra.

Brown, M., Grbich, C., Maddocks, I., Parker, D., Roe, P. & Willis, E. (2005). Documenting end of life decisions in residential aged care facilities in South Australia. *Australian and New Zealand Journal of Public Health, 29*(1), 85–90.

Detering, K., Hancock, A., Reade, M. & Silvester, W. (2010). The impact of advance care planning on end of life care in elderly patients: Randomised controlled trial. *British Medical Journal*, 340, 1345. doi: 10.1136/bmj.c1345

Government of Western Australia. (2010). *A Guide to Enduring Power of Guardianship in Western Australia*. Perth.

Hammes, B. & Rooney, B. (1998). Death and end-of-life planning in one midwestern community. *Archives of Internal Medicine*, 158, 383–90.

Ministry of Health New Zealand. (2011). *Advance Care Planning: A guide for the New Zealand health care workforce*. Wellington.

Nair, B., Kerridge, I., Dobson, A., McPhee, J. & Saul, P. (2000). Advance care planning in residential aged care. *Australian and New Zealand Journal of Medicine*, 30, 339–43.

Parker, D., Hughes, K. & Tuckett, A. (2011). *Implementing and Evaluating a Comprehensive Model of Palliative Care in Residential Aged Care Facilities. Report to Department of Health and Ageing*. Brisbane: University of Queensland.

Shanley, C., Whitmore, E., Khoo, A., Cartright, C., Walker, A. & Cumming, R. (2009). Understanding how advance care planning is approached in the residential aged care setting: A continuum model of practice as an explanatory device. *Australasian Journal of Ageing*, 28(4), 211–15.

Silvester, W., Parslow, R., Lewis, V., Fullam, R., Sjanta, R., Jackson, L.,...Hudson, R. (2013). Development and evaluation of an aged care specific Advance Care Plan. *BMJ Supportive and Palliative Care*, 3, 188–95.

Street, A. & Ottman, G. (2006). *State of the Science Review of Advance Care Planning Models*. Bundoora: LaTrobe University.

University of Queensland. (2012). *The Palliative Approach Toolkit Module 2 – Key Processes*. Brisbane: University of Queensland.

12 A strengths-based palliative approach for the frail older adult living in residential aged care

Deborah Parker

Learning objectives

After reading this chapter you will be able to:

1 Have an understanding of a palliative approach in residential aged care.

2 Understand the key features of an evidence-based palliative approach in residential aged care.

3 Understand how to apply a strengths-based approach to a palliative approach for people living in residential aged care.

4 Understand specific issues in providing a palliative approach for people with dementia.

Introduction

This chapter extends some of the issues introduced to you in Chapter 10 which identified a model of palliative care that has been developed specifically for Australian residential aged care facilities (RACFs). This comprehensive evidence-based model of a palliative approach in residential aged care is encapsulated in an evidence translation product known as the Palliative Approach Toolkit (Parker, Hughes & Tuckett, 2011). Before we explore this model of care we will briefly review some of the research and issues specific to providing a palliative approach in RACFs. The final section of the chapter will identify some specific issues for people with dementia in RACF and some programs that have been developed to address these.

A palliative approach in residential aged care facilities

Researchers and clinicians both internationally and in Australia have had a long interest in the interface between palliative care and residential aged care. An early study from South Australia (Maddocks et al., 1996) provided the most comprehensive picture of palliative care in residential aged care in Australia. The findings suggested the need for better assessment and treatment of pain for residents with dementia, more comprehensive advance care planning (ACP), education for all staff including general practitioners and increased liaison between RACFs and palliative care services.

Following this an intervention study in residential aged care was conducted (Maddocks et al., 1999). This study provided the opportunity for RACFs within the southern region of Adelaide the opportunity to appoint 'link nurses' who received training to become the key palliative care supports within their organisation. For an additional six month period, two **palliative care clinical nurse consultants** provided specific support for on-site education and clinical consultations. Staff evaluated these interventions positively and reported improved outcomes for residents.

Palliative care clinical nurse consultants
Registered nurses with specialist knowledge in palliative care.

A follow-up study by these investigators (Grbich et al., 2003) specifically focused on the palliative care needs of residents with a non-cancer diagnosis. Conducted approximately eight years after the national palliative care study, the results from Maddocks et al. (1996) indicated that almost two thirds of RACFs in South Australia do access specialist palliative care services for education and clinical consultation. While many of the issues raised during the 1996 study showed improvement there was still little uniformity across these institutions concerning ACP and few residents had advance directives in place.

Palliative care case conferences
Multidisciplinary meetings with the resident, family, general practitioner and nursing care team. The focus is on palliative and end of life care.

An important initiative in Australia, already discussed in Chapter 10, was the development of multidisciplinary palliative care guidelines specifically for RACFs (Commonwealth of Australia, 2006). The first study using these guidelines to form the basis of care was conducted by Abbey, Sacre and Parker (2008). The model of care used in this study in two residential aged care settings in Australia included education for all staff and the use of **palliative care case conferences** and care planning. The model of care was evaluated using a pre- and post-study design; that is, care was compared for 25 residents prior to the implementation of the model with care for 17 residents who received the model of care. Outcomes were measured by chart audits, the Symptom Management at the End-of-Life in Dementia (SM-EOLD) and the Satisfaction with Care at the End-of-Life in Dementia (SWC-EOLD) Scales (Volicer, Hurley & Blasi, 2001). The main findings were that the use of palliative care case conferencing increased from 12 to 71 per cent and that there was a slight increase in the use of advance health directives (8% to 12%). However, documentation of the occurrence of all symptoms using the SM-EOLD increased. This was most probably due to the focus in the education sessions on the importance of assessment and documentation rather than a decrease in care that would indicate greater symptom burden. Carer satisfaction using the SWC-EOLD increased slightly for carers whose family members received the new model of care (mean 30.68 pre and mean 31 post). The authors concluded that providing a structured multidisciplinary approach for residents with end stage dementia shows some promising results but more work in this area is required.

In the UK the promotion of a standardised model of care using the **Gold Standards Framework** (GSF) has seen improvements across a range of settings including long-term care. The GSF includes a process of identifying those in the final year or so of life and their stage of illness, assessing what they need and implementing good communication to achieve those goals. Key tasks are designed to improve end of life care based on the 7 Cs – communication, coordination, control of symptoms, continuity, continued learning, carer support and care of the dying. Residents are classified using a needs-based coding system whereby people are assigned as 'stable' (year plus **prognosis**), 'unstable or advanced disease' (month's prognosis), 'deteriorating' (week's prognosis),' final days or terminal care' and 'after care'. Badger et al. (2009) reports on the evaluation of 49 long-term care homes that completed pre- and post-evaluation surveys of the use of the GSF. Following the implementation of the GSF long-term care homes were more likely to have a register for end of life care, a coordinator for end of life care, discussions regarding cardiopulmonary resuscitation, were able to meet the residents' spiritual needs, provide better quality of care to residents, supporting family carers and quality of support for staff. While the GSF is popular in the UK and forms part of their end of life care strategy, there has been only limited use of GSF in Australia. This is primarily because there is a fee for use of the GSF (Gold Standards Framework, 2013).

Gold Standards Framework
A model of palliative care used in the UK across a range of settings including long-term care.

Prognosis
Includes the expected duration, function and a description of the course of the disease.

An evidence-based palliative approach: what are the key features and does it work?

In Australia a comprehensive evidence-based model of care has been developed and evaluated (Parker, Hughes & Tuckett, 2011). Like the GSF residents are categorised based on needs using estimated prognosis as a trigger. In this model there are three trajectories and three key processes linked to each of these trajectories (Figure 12.1). The Palliative Approach Toolkit provides extensive educational and training products to implement the model. This includes information on how to undertake the three key processes – **advance care planning**, conducting a palliative care case conference and using an **end of life care pathway**. A focus on five common symptoms – which include pain, dyspnoea, nutrition and hydration, oral care and delirium – is also provided.

The following short overview of each trajectory will indicate how key processes are incorporated as part of the model. In trajectory 'A' residents have an estimated prognosis of greater than six months. All new and existing residents should have the opportunity to express their wishes about ACP and have these clearly documented in their case notes. We have already discussed ACP in Chapter 11. Remember ACP is the process of communication between a competent resident and the person's health care team. It does not have to be a legalised formal process but it may result in the completion of an **advance care directive** (ACD). Residents on this trajectory of care should be reviewed every six months or sooner if there is a significant change that suggests a prognosis of six months or less.

Residents in trajectory 'B' have an estimated prognosis of six months or less. The key process in this trajectory is to conduct a palliative care case conference. A palliative care case conference (PCC) is a meeting held between a resident (and/or their family) and their care providers. The aims of a PCC are to identify clear goals of care for the resident including a review of any advance care plans. It also provides a safe environment where issues and questions about end of life care can be raised and appropriate

Advance care planning
A process whereby a person's values, beliefs and preferences are made known so that they can be used to guide decision making in circumstances where the person is no longer able to do so.

End of life care pathway
A structured document that focuses on care required in the last few days or week of life.

Advance care directive A legal document that sets out instructions that consent to or refuse specified medical treatments. It is designed to be enacted when the person is no longer able to make informed decisions.

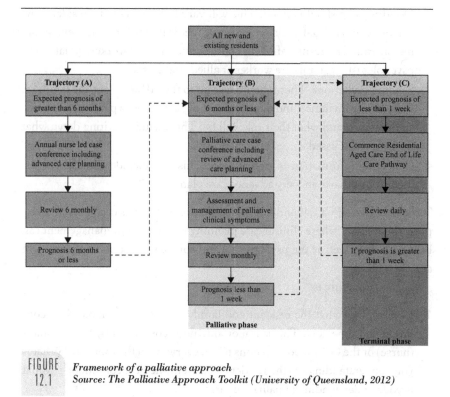

FIGURE 12.1   *Framework of a palliative approach*
Source: The Palliative Approach Toolkit (University of Queensland, 2012)

strategies agreed upon. The effectiveness of PCCs for patients receiving care from specialist palliative care services has demonstrated benefits such as improved quality of life (Mitchell et al., 2005), maintenance of function (Mitchell, Tieman & Shelby-James, 2008; Shelby-James et al., 2012), significant reduction in hospitalisations (Mitchell et al., 2008), increased coordination of care (Mitchell et al., 2005; Shelby-James et al., 2007) and information transfer (Mitchell et al., 2005; Mitchell et al., 2002).

Palliative care case conferences

In the Palliative Approach Toolkit tips and strategies for planning a PCC are provided at: www.caresearch.com.au/PAToolkit. In summary these include:

1   Deciding who should facilitate a PCC. It can be convened and facilitated by a registered nurse from the RACF or the resident's general practitioner (GP).

2   Deciding who should attend. This will vary but it can be the resident, the person who has legal decision maker or medical power of attorney, family members and relevant staff. This could include a social worker, geriatrician, psychologist, pastoral care worker or allied health staff.

3   Sending invitations. These should be sent to the GP as well as the family. A PCC family invitation and questionnaire explains what a palliative care case conference is and what their role will be. This includes writing down what they want discussed.

4   Collecting information in preparation. This will include clinical records, medication charts and any advance care plans.

To be effective a PCC should follow a structure that allows each person to express their views, where clinical care planning and symptom management can be discussed as well as the psychosocial and spiritual concerns of the resident and their family.

A good structure is:

1   Determining what the resident and family already know about their condition and trajectory. This is important and is conducted by the facilitator (nurse) or the GP. Good questions to ask everyone in the room are 'What is your understanding of (the resident's) current medical condition?'; 'What is your understanding of palliative care?'

2   Ascertaining what changes have occurred in terms of functional decline, weight loss, recent hospital admissions, changes to medications or other clinical care These will indicate if they are in trajectory 'B' (less than six months to live).

3   Reviewing the person's current status, prognosis and treatment options. Be careful to take into account the preferences of the resident and family regarding how much they wish to be told.

4   Asking the resident and family in turn if they have any questions about current status, prognosis and treatment options. Review the family questionnaire if completed.

5   Exploring what decisions about the resident's care that the resident (if present) or the family need to consider. These may be regarding clinical care or lifestyle.

6   Providing a summary of what was covered including any decisions and actions at the end of the PCC.

7 Documenting what was discussed in the person's case notes. Amend the resident's care plan to reflect outcomes and action plans.

Following the PCC the care plan should be reviewed each month and adjusted as the resident's care needs change utilising the domains of care as appropriate. If the resident has signs and symptoms that suggested that they may die within the next week (require terminal care) they are in trajectory 'C' and end of life care pathway should be commenced. The Residential Aged Care End of Life Care Pathway (RAC EoLCP) has been developed and evaluated positively in Australian RACFs. The use of this pathway reduces unnecessary hospital admissions and improves terminal care (Reymond, Israel & Charles, 2011).

The effectiveness of this model of care was demonstrated in a study of nine RACFs. Using a pre- and post-test design, the care of 84 residents before the model was introduced was compared to the care provided for 73 residents where care was directed using the model described. The study demonstrated improvements in the clinical care of residents such as symptom management, communication with families, advance care planning, bereavement care, referrals to specialist services (palliative care, pain management) and care in the final days of life. There were significant increases between the pre- to post-intervention in documented evidence on the initial admission form for any information regarding end of life wishes (55.4% compared to 72.6%), documented evidence that relatives or legal guardians were involved in end of life discussions (71.1% compared to 95.7%) and care matching wishes on advance care plan (82.6% compared to 95.5%). Uptake of PCCs was high for the intervention group (94.5% compared to 8.4% in the pre-intervention group). Of the 42 residents who died in the data collection period, 28 (66.7%) were commenced on the RAC EoLCP (Parker, Hughes & Tuckett, 2011).

You will recall in Chapter 10 that we discussed the strengths-based approach to palliative care. While this was not specific to RACF the tenets outlined in Table 10.1 (p. 162) are relevant to the model previously described by Parker, Hughes and Tuckett (2011). The tenet of self-determination of the resident is facilitated by the key process of advance care planning (discussed in the case scenario in Chapter 10) and the tenets of empowerment, collaboration and regeneration are all present in the key process PCC and using an end of life care pathway.

Using a strengths-based approach to palliative care

We have followed Beryl through her journey in the last two chapters. When we first met Beryl she was living alone in her own home and receiving care as part of a Home Care Package.

Beryl has now been living in the local residential aged care facility for six months but has had a number of admissions to hospital due to her heart failure and on each admission she does not recover to the same level as prior to her hospitalisation.

In the case scenario in Chapter 10 we discussed advance care planning for Beryl. As Beryl has become increasingly frail she has entered into trajectory 'B' on the palliative care model described in this chapter. A palliative care case conference is required to discuss her clinical care and end of life wishes with her and her family.

Reflective questions

You are the registered nurse looking after Beryl and have to arrange a PCC.

› How do you go about organising it?

› Who would you invite?

› How will you know what the family wants to discuss?

› What are some of the outcomes that you think might arise from a PCC?

Reflective activity

Reflect on an older person you have cared for whom you considered to be in trajectory 'B'.

● What processes occurred that facilitated discussions about end of life care? If this did not occur, why not?

● How confident would you be to participate or convene a PCC?

● What are some of the skills you might require to effectively conduct a PCC?

● What gaps in your knowledge have you identified that you could fill by further reading or education?

Dementia specific initiatives in providing palliative care

There is limited evidence to date of the efficacy of specific interventions of a palliative approach for people with advanced dementia. While the model described in the previous section has been evaluated for people with dementia it is not a dementia specific palliative care model. Several literature reviews have examined the main issues for providing end of life care for people with dementia

(Birch & Draper, 2008; Volicer, 2008). In the Volicer review this concerned cardiopulmonary resuscitation, transfers to an acute setting, infections, nutritional issues, decisions about end of life care and hospice care. Recommendations from the review included that: (i) cardiopulmonary resuscitation should only be performed if specifically requested by the person or their surrogate; (ii) maintenance of oral health decreases the incidence of pneumonia; (iii) antibiotics should not be routinely prescribed for generalised infections but comfort should be maintained; (iv) discussions concerning end of life care should be occur soon after admission to RACF and physicians should be encouraged to be involved in these discussions. In the review by Birch and Draper (2008), four key themes were identified: (i) difficulties associated with diagnosing the terminal phase of the illness (prognostication); (ii) issues relating to communication; (iii) medical interventions and (iv) the appropriateness of palliative care interventions.

A study currently being conducted in Australia is the Integrated Care Framework for Advanced Dementia (ICF-D), which is a framework to guide point-of-care palliative dementia care (http://icfdementia.org/). It includes a suite of web-based interactive resources incorporating an online assessment tool, care plans based on individual assessments to enable person-centred care, communication guides with associated family fact sheets, education modules for staff and audiovisual teaching materials, and an audit and reporting tool. At present no evaluation reports are available for this project.

Namaste Care™

Namaste Care™ was developed in the US and provides residents with dementia and their families with quality care that addresses not only physical but also emotional and spiritual needs (Simard, 2013; Simard & Volicer, 2010). It is designed as a seven day a week program in which specifically trained care assistants provide 'high touch low tech' interventions in a specifically designed room. A trial of this program was conducted in four long-term care settings (Simard & Volicer, 2010). The rooms had low lighting, soft relaxing music and the use of aromatherapy such as lavender to promote relaxation. The focus of the activities, provided by the care assistant, was around activities of daily living. For example, clipping fingernails is a task done after the completion of a shower or bath often in a hurried manner by a care assistant eager to move through the list of tasks. In the Namaste program, the care assistant performed this activity in a slow and deliberate manner. Residents had their hands soaked in a warm

Namaste Care™ A program of person-centred care for people with dementia.

lavender scented basin. This was often combined for women with having their face washed and moisturised. The aim of the program was to provide pleasant stimuli for residents. This included residents being offered regular pleasant drinks, listening to soothing music, such as rainforest sounds, and being able to touch or discuss objects relevant to the season.

In this trial (Simard & Volicer, 2010) Namaste Care[TM] was provided for approximately five hours per day for 86 residents with dementia with each group having between six and 11 residents in the Namaste room with at least one care assistant. Outcome measures included depression, delirium indicators and behaviour. There was no difference in depression scores before and after the trial; however, only eight residents had a baseline score that would indicate that they had depression. There were also no significant differences between behavioural symptoms before and after enrolment in the whole study population. However, for a sub-group analysis of residents with reduced social interaction, the Namaste Program did increase social interaction and there was a trend for decreased agitation and delirium.

A study focusing specifically on 37 residents with end stage dementia was conducted at six care homes in the UK (Stacpoole et al., 2004). Results indicated that in care homes with good pain management, Namaste Care[TM] was significantly effective in reducing behavioural symptom severity over time and this reduction was not related to increased analgesia. Both of these studies indicate promising results for the use of Namaste Care[TM] for people with dementia including those

A palliative approach to dementia

Case scenario 12.2

Jo is an 85 year old man who has been in an RACF for three years. He lived for most of his life on a small fruit and vegetable farm. His wife died 10 years ago and, when he was diagnosed with Alzheimer's disease five years ago, he and his two daughters made the decision for him to relocate from the family farm into care.

Jo's condition has steadily deteriorated over the last three years. He still recognises family members sometimes when they visit. In the last few months Jo has become increasingly annoyed with staff members and paces around the dementia specific unit looking for an exit to the garden. Jo is considered to be in trajectory 'A' as,

despite having Alzheimer's for five years, he is still physically well and stable.

Reflective questions

You are the registered nurse looking after Jo and have been asked to work with his daughters and the diversional therapist to come up with a program of activities that will decrease his unsettled behaviour.

Review the ROPES assessment model described in Chapter 3 (pp. 43–4).

> Using this model and the strength-based approach, what activities are most suitable for Jo?

> How will you know if these activities have been successful in making Jo feel valued as a person?

who are dying. However, costing for the sustainability of this program is required before it can be adopted as standard practice across Australia and New Zealand.

Summary

- A model of a palliative approach in residential aged care can improve the end of life care provided to older people.
- Conducting a palliative care case conference will assist you in providing a strengths-based approach for people living in residential aged care who have a life limiting illness.
- A palliative approach for people with dementia can be facilitated by programs that build on the strengths of the person.

Conclusion

This chapter has provided an overview of an evidence-based model of palliative care for use in residential aged care facilities that aligns with the strengths-based approach used in this book. Using the key processes within the model an individual's needs can be ascertained and good communication facilitated throughout the person's trajectory. For residents with dementia, programs that build on the person's life biography can improve quality of life and decrease behavioural symptoms.

Further reading

You may like to take a look at the following reading recommendation: Caresearch at http://www.caresearch.com.au

References

Abbey, J., Sacre, S. & Parker, D. (2008). *Develop, Trial and Evaluate a Model of Multidisciplinary Palliative Care for Residents with End-stage Dementia*. Brisbane: Queensland University of Technology.

Badger, F., Clifford, C., Hewison, A. & Thomas, K. (2009). An evaluation of the implementation of a programme to improve end-of-life care in nursing homes. *Palliative Medicine*, 23, 502–11.

Birch, D. & Draper, J. (2008). A critical literature review exploring the challenges of delivering effective palliative care to older people with dementia. *Journal of Clinical Nursing*, 17, 1144–63.

Commonwealth of Australia. (2006). *Guidelines for a Palliative Approach in Residential Aged Care Facilities – NHMRC Endorsed Edition*. Canberra. Retrieved from http://www.nhmrc.gov.au/publications/synopses/ac12to14syn.htm

Gold Standards Framework. (2013). Retrieved from http://www.goldstandardsframework.org.uk/index.html

Grbich, C., Maddocks, I., Parker, D., Piller, N., Brown, M., Willis, E., Connellan, P. & Hofmeyer, A. (2003). *Palliative Care in Residential Aged Care Facilities for Residents with Non-Cancer Diagnosis. Reports to the NHMRC*. Adelaide: Flinders University.

Maddocks, I., Abbey, J., Pickhaver, A., Parker, D., Beck, K. & DeBellis, A. (1996). *Palliative Care in Nursing Homes. Report to the Commonwealth Department of Health and Family Services*. Adelaide: Flinders University.

Maddocks, I., Parker, D., McLeod, A. & Jenkin, P. (1999). *Palliative Care Nurse Practitioners in Aged Care Facilities. Report to the Department of Human Services, South Australian Government*. Adelaide: International Institute of Hospice Studies.

Mitchell, G., Cherry, M., Kennedy, R., Burridge, L. & Clavarion, A. (2005). General practitioner, specialist providers case conferences in palliative care: Lessons learned from 56 case conferences. *Australian Family Physician*, 34(5), 389–92.

Mitchell, G., Del Mar, C., Clavarino, A., de Jong, I. & Kennedy, R. (2002). General practitioner attitudes to case conferences: How can we increase participation and effectiveness? *Medical Journal of Australia*, 177, 95–7.

Mitchell, G., Tieman, J. & Shelby-James, T. (2008). Multidisciplinary care planning and teamwork in primary care. *The Medical Journal of Australia*. 188(8 Suppl), S61–S64.

Parker, D., Hughes, K. & Tuckett, A. (2011). *Implementing and Evaluating a Comprehensive Model of Palliative Care in Residential Aged Care Facilities. Report to Department of Health and Ageing*. Brisbane: University of Queensland.

Reymond, L., Israel, F. & Charles, M. (2011). A residential aged care end-of-life care pathway (RAC EoLCP) for Australian aged care facilities. *Australian Health Review*, 35(3). doi: 10.1071/AH10899

Shelby-James, T., Butow, P., Davison, G. & Currow, D. (2012). Case conferences in palliative care. A substudy of a cluster randomised controlled trial. *Australian Family Physician*, 41(8), 608–12.

Shelby-James, T., Currow, D., Phillips, J., Williams, H. & Abernethy, A. (2007). Promoting patient centred palliative care through case conferencing. *Australian Family Physician*, 36(11), 961–4.

Simard, J. (2013). *The End-of-Life Namaste Care Program for People with Dementia*. Baltimore: Health Professions Press Inc.

Simard, J. & Volicer, L. (2010). Effects of Namaste Care^{TM} on residents who do not benefit from usual activities. *American Journal of Alzheimer's Disease and Other Dementias*, 25(1), 46–50.

Stacpoole, M., Thompsell, A., Hockley, J., Simard, J. & Volicer, L. (2004). *Implementing the Namaste Care Programme for People with Advanced Dementia at the End of Their Lives: An Action Research Study in Six Care Homes with Nursing.* London: St Christopher's Hospice.

University of Queensland. (2012). *The Palliative Approach Toolkit Module 2 – Key Processes.* Brisbane.

Volicer, L. (2008). End-of-life care for people with dementia in long-term care settings. *Alzheimer's Care Today,* 9(2), 84–102.

Volicer, L., Hurley, A.C. & Blasi, Z.V. (2001). Scales for evaluation of end-of-life care in dementia. *Alzheimer Disease & Associated Disorders,* 15(4), 194–200.

Evidence-based nursing interventions: a good death and fostering pain relief

13

Deborah Parker

Learning objectives

After reading this chapter you will be able to:

1   Have an understanding of what constitutes a 'good death' for older people.

2   Understand the principles of evidence-based nursing in relation to pain assessment and management.

3   Understand specific issues in the assessment and management of pain for people with dementia.

4   Understand how to apply a strengths-based approach to pain assessment and management for older people.

Introduction

In Chapter 10 we reviewed the history of palliative care with specific reference to developments in Australia and New Zealand. Chapter 11 focused on advance care planning, which is a critical aspect of providing a strengths-based palliative approach for older people. Chapter 12 specifically looked at some of the research regarding providing a palliative approach in residential aged care facilities (RACFs) and the evidence-based model within the Palliative Approach Toolkit. This chapter delves further into what makes a good death for older people and then specifically focuses on one common symptom that can influence whether a good death is possible – pain. Pain is one of the most common symptoms and always features in discussions with people who know they are dying, families supporting that person or staff providing the care. The phrase most associated with achieving a good death is that it is 'pain free'. In the final section of the chapter we will examine specific issues in regard to pain management and people with dementia.

What makes a good death?

In Chapter 10, the definition of palliative care was reviewed. To recap, this included addressing quality of life of people with a life limiting illness by identifying and managing a person's physical, psychosocial and spiritual issues and their families (World Health Organization, 2014). While this definition is useful to understand the holistic approach that palliative care encompasses it does not specify what makes a good death. An early definition by Field and Cassel (1997) is that a good death is free from avoidable distress and suffering for patients, families and caregivers; in general accord with patients' and families' wishes; and reasonably consistent with clinical, cultural and ethical standards.

More recent explorations of differing views on what constitutes a good death are reported in the literature. Steinhauser et al. (2000) conducted a study in the US convening focus groups with a range of people involved in end of life care including physicians, nurses, social workers, chaplains, hospice volunteers, patients and recently bereaved family members. These groups identified six major components of a good death:

1 Pain and symptom management.
2 Clear decision making.
3 Preparation for death including what to expect as death approaches.
4 Completion, which includes spiritual issues, life review, resolving conflicts, spending time with family and friends, and saying goodbye.
5 Contributing to others which may be provision of gifts, time or knowledge.
6 Affirmation of the whole person as unique.

In this study there were differences between what dying people, their families and providers identified as a good death although all six themes were present for patients, families and non-physician health care providers. The physicians by contrast had a more biomedical view than any other groups and they did not identify the theme 'contributing to others'.

A study in the UK by Lloyd-Williams et al. (2007) provides a unique older person's view. In this study they interviewed 40 older people living alone in the community. Six key themes were identified by these individuals:

1 Fears related to end of life.
2 The inevitability of death.
3 Thoughts and wishes related to end of life care.
4 Preparations for end of life.
5 **Euthanasia**/assisted dying.
6 Thoughts regarding an afterlife.

While there are many similarities between these themes and those identified by Steinhauser et al. (2000), the focus from older people is much more on the individual's role in their dying. Specific in this study was the fear related to end of life which included concern about dying at home alone, and existential issues such as assisted dying and the afterlife. These differences may have occurred as the sample in this study were those aged 80 years and over living in the community, however they were not terminally ill or receiving end of life services.

> **Euthanasia** The act of deliberately ending the life of a patient for the purpose of ending intolerable pain and/or suffering.

The most comprehensive list specifically related to the care of older people dying is proposed by the Age Health and Care Study Group in the UK and reported by Smith (2000) as follows:

1 To know when death is coming and to understand what can be expected.
2 To be able to retain control of what happens.
3 To be afforded dignity and privacy.
4 To have control over pain relief and other symptom control.
5 To have choice and control over where death occurs (at home or elsewhere).
6 To have access to information and expertise of whatever kind is necessary.
7 To have access to any spiritual or emotional support required.
8 To have access to hospice care in any location, not only in hospital.
9 To have control over who is present and who shares the end.
10 To be able to issue advance directives which ensure wishes are respected.
11 To have time to say goodbye and control over other aspects of timing.
12 To be able to leave when it is time to go and not to have life prolonged pointlessly.

These 12 issues reflect both those of the health professionals and consumers raised by the previous studies. It is a very comprehensive summary and the language used reflects the strengths-based approach that we advocate throughout the book – in particular 'choice' and 'control'.

Evidence-based practice: pain assessment and management

Pain is an unpleasant sensory and emotional experience associated with actual or potential tissue damage or more simply, pain is a subjective experience, occurring when and where the person says it does (Turk & Melzack, 1992). The prevalence of reported pain in older people varies widely. Fox, Raina and Jada (1999), in a systematic review of pain in older people in RACFs, identified six studies where prevalence of pain was reported by direct measure. In these studies self-reported pain was estimated as 49 to 83 per cent with musculoskeletal pain the most common. In a further five studies, where analgesic use was used as a proxy for prevalence of pain, these figures are significantly less – 27 to 44 per cent. Prevalence of pain within community dwelling older adults is not widely reported. In a study of older Australians randomly selected from electoral rolls, chronic pain prevalence was 51 per cent in the 65–74 year age group and 55 per cent for those aged 85 years and over (Helme & Gibson, 1999). A study by Blyth et al. (2001) using the New South Wales Health Survey population found that prevalence of chronic pain peaked for males at 27.0 per cent in the 65–69 year age group and for females, prevalence peaked at 31.0 per cent in the oldest age group (80–84 years). From these reports we can see that pain is a common symptom for older people although it is not only confined to those who require palliative care. However, when reviewing the elements of a good death, in each of the three studies cited being free from pain was one of the good death criteria. In this section of the chapter we explore pain in more detail and specifically examine the best evidence for pain assessment and management.

Assessing pain

A thorough pain assessment is important. The Australian Pain Society (2005) identifies eight factors that should be considered in completing a comprehensive pain assessment.

These are:

1 A thorough pain history including when the pain began, severity, relieving factors and where the pain occurs.
2 General medical history such as relevant diseases that will impact on pain and any associated symptoms.

3 Physical examination which includes site and referred pain, presence of arthritis and sensory changes.

4 Physical impact of the pain on activities of daily living, movement or activity and functional assessment.

5 Psychosocial situation which may impact on pain such as the person's coping resources, beliefs about pain, mental health issues and family expectations or beliefs about pain.

6 Social impact of pain in regard to relationships and social activities.

7 Review of medications and treatments.

8 Prognosis.

Valid and reliable pain assessment tools should be used to assist in this comprehensive assessment of pain for the older adult. The Australian Pain Society (2005) recommends five pain assessment tools for use in RACFs. These scales are also suitable for older people living in the community. Three of these are for people able to communicate and two for people with dementia. The three scales for people able to communicate are:

1 The Modified Residents' Verbal Brief Pain Inventory (M-RVBPI).

2 A numeric rating scale.

3 A verbal descriptor scale.

The M-RVBPI should be used for an initial pain assessment and for periodic reviews. It provides a comprehensive overview of the resident's pain and covers many of the factors previously discussed. For ongoing pain assessment a one-dimensional pain assessment instrument such as a numeric rating scale or verbal descriptor scale is most appropriate. Numeric rating scales involve asking the patient to rate their pain from 0 to 10, with 0 representing one end of the pain continuum (for example, no pain) and 10 representing the other extreme of pain intensity (for example, pain as bad as it could be). A verbal descriptor scale consists of a series of phrases that represent different levels of pain intensity (for example, 'no pain', 'mild pain', 'moderate pain', 'severe pain', 'extreme pain', and 'the most intense pain imaginable') (Herr & Garand, 2001). Pain may be more pronounced or only occur when a person moves or is moved. A thorough assessment should include a movement-based protocol; that is, getting the person, if able, to move independently and report pain on movement. If the person is not able to move independently gently raising their arms or standing or walking (if not contraindicated) is recommended or if the person is not mobile moving the person in the bed is useful. The pain assessment of people with dementia is addressed in a later section of this chapter.

Treatment of pain

Pain management should include pharmacological and non-pharmacological options. Critical to an effective pain management plan is that the type of pain should be identified. The two main pain types are **nociceptive** or **neuropathic pain**. Nociceptive pain occurs as a result of the stimulation of nerve endings in skin and deep tissue. Nociceptive pain is further classified into three different types according to the stimulus – superficial somatic, somatic and visceral (see Table 13.1 for further details). Neuropathic pain occurs when nerves are damaged.

Nociceptive pain This is caused by the stimulation of nerve endings in skin and deep tissue.
Neuropathic pain This is caused by damage to nerves.

Pharmacological treatment will depend on the type and the severity of pain. Mild pain is usually controlled by paracetamol or non-steroidal anti-inflammatory drugs (NSAIDs). Opioids may be required for more severe pain but can also be combined with paracetamol or NSAIDs. Neuropathic pain may not respond completely to opioids (Therapeutic Guidelines, 2010). Non-pharmacological approaches to pain management include application of heat or cold, mild vibration, massage, complementary therapies,

TABLE 13.1 *Classification of pain*

	NOCICEPTIVE SUPERFICIAL SOMATIC	NOCICEPTIVE DEEP SOMATIC	NOCICEPTIVE VISCERAL	NEUROPATHIC
Stimulus	Skin, subcutaneous tissue	Bones, muscles, organ capsules	Solid or hollow organs, lymph nodes or tumour masses	Damage to autonomic nerves and nociceptive pathways
Examples	Stomatitis	Fractures	Abdominal masses or colic	Neuralgia or nerve pain due to a tumour
Description	Hot, sharp, stinging pain	Dull, aching or throbbing pain	Dull, cramping or colicky pain	Pins and needles, burning or shooting pain
Pharmacological treatment options	Paracetamol Corticosteroids NSAIDs Opioids	NSAIDs Opioids Baclofen	Paracetamol Corticosteroids Opioids Ketamine Anti-spasmodics	Opioids Anti-epileptic Corticosteroids
Non-pharmacological treatment options	Heat or cold Immobilisation	Massage Heat or cold	Heat or cold	

Source: Adapted from Therapeutic Guidelines, 2005

relaxation, guiding imagery, cognitive behavioural strategies and the use of transcutaneous electrical nerve stimulation (Australian Pain Society, 2005). Table 13.1 has some characteristics of the different pain types and examples of non-pharmacological and pharmacological treatment options.

Pain assessment and management for people with dementia

A systematic review by McAuliffe et al. (2009) sought to identify barriers to pain assessment and strategies to overcome these barriers for people with dementia. Main barriers to pain assessment were lack of recognition of pain, insufficient education, misdiagnosis and non-use of assessment tools.

Extensive research into appropriate pain assessment tools for people with dementia has been conducted and there are six common behavioural indicators that are useful in identifying possible presence of pain for people with dementia (Herr, Bjoro & Decker, 2006). These are:

1 *Facial expressions*: slight frown, sad, frightened face, grimacing, wrinkled forehead, closed or tightened eyes, any distorted expression, rapid blinking.
2 *Verbalisations, vocalisations*: sighing, moaning, groaning, grunting, chanting, calling out, noisy breathing, asking for help.
3 *Body movements*: rigid, tense body posture, guarding, fidgeting increased pacing, rocking, restricted movement, gait or mobility changes.
4 *Changes in interpersonal interactions*: aggressive, combative, resisting care, decreased social interactions, socially inappropriate, disruptive, withdrawn, and verbally abusive.
5 *Changes in activity patterns or routines*: refusing food, appetite change, increase in rest periods or sleep, changes in rest pattern, sudden cessation of common routines, increased wandering.
6 *Mental status changes*: crying or tears, increased confusion, irritability or distress.

The Australian Pain Society (2005) recommends two pain scales for use with people with dementia and both include these common behavioural indicators:

1 The Abbey Pain Scale (Abbey et al., 2004).
2 The Pain Assessment in Advanced Dementia (PAINAD) Scale (Warden, Hurley & Volicer, 2003).

The Abbey Scale is an Australian tool developed to measure intensity of pain in people with late stage dementia. The tool includes six items: vocalisation, facial expression, change in body language, behavioural change, physiological change and physical change. Each item is scored on a 4-point scale for intensity of the behaviour (absent = 0, mild = 1, moderate = 2, severe = 3) with total score ranging from 0 to 18. The total score is then interpreted as intensity of pain: no pain = 0–2, mild = 3–7, moderate = 8–13, and severe = 14+. The person rating is asked to indicate which type of pain the older adult has: **chronic**, **acute**, or **acute on chronic**.

> **Chronic pain** Pain that has lasted longer than three to six months and does not resolve in response to treatment.

Similarly to people without dementia it is important when conducting a pain assessment for someone with dementia to use a movement-based protocol. In some instances people with dementia will stop wandering or have a decrease in their behaviours (less calling out) and this can be due to unrecognised pain. It is therefore important to know what is usual for the person by having a good behavioural assessment as well as pain assessment. Copies of both the Abbey and the PAINAD are available in the Australian Pain Society management strategies booklet (Australian Pain Society, 2005).

> **Acute pain** The body's normal response to damage such as a cut, an infection or other physical injuries. This type of pain usually comes on fast and often goes away in no more than a few weeks or months if treated properly.

Pain management for people with dementia should be the same as that described for people who are still able to communicate in that it will require pharmacological and non-pharmacological options. However, as it is difficult if not impossible for people with dementia to verbally report to the assessor the effect of pain interventions, what is crucially important is a reassessment of the person's pain using a valid and reliable tool such as those identified.

> **Acute on chronic pain** Pain that is between acute and chronic, and may also be known as subacute pain.

Strengths-based pain management

As you will have seen in this chapter pain is a complex symptom that will require good assessment using valid and reliable pain assessment tools. However, there are many other factors that will influence how a person experiences or manages their pain that are not easily incorporated into a standardised pain assessment tool. In Chapter 3 you were introduced to the ROPES Assessment Model (Graybeal, 2001). Remember this acronym stands for '**R**esources, **O**pportunities, **P**ossibilities, **E**xceptions and **S**olutions'. Let's revisit this model and how it might be applied when assessing a person's pain in Table 13.2.

TABLE 13.2 *ROPES Assessment Model*

Resources	What personal, family, social, organisational and community resources does the patient have?	Pain can be impacted upon by the person's psychosocial, social and spiritual needs. Understanding what resources the person has may help mitigate these impacts.
Options	What options are available in terms of focus and choice?	Pain management is not only pharmacological management. Identify with the person what other options they would like to try in regard to non-pharmacological managements and alternative therapies.
Possibilities	What possibilities are available in terms of the patient's future. What has been thought of but not tried?	Similar to options, identify what other possibilities in regard to management strategies are available and acceptable to the person.
Exceptions	When is the problem not happening? When is the problem different?	A further pain assessment will identify triggers as well as things that ameliorate the pain.
Solutions	Ask 'What's working now?' What are the successes? What would the patient like to continue?	Pain management strategies must be tailored to the individual.

A strengths-based approach to pain

Case scenario 13.1

We have followed Beryl through her journey in the last three chapters. When we first met Beryl she was living alone in her own home. Beryl is 85, has end stage heart failure, non-insulin dependent diabetes, osteoarthritis and cataracts. Beryl had been living at home receiving a Home Care Package but as she became increasingly frail she moved into the local residential aged care facility. Beryl has a clear palliative care plan from her case conference but recently her pain from her osteoarthritis has been bothering her. She complains to her daughters that she is in so much pain that it is hard for her to move around freely and it is really impacting on her quality of life. She is currently on regular paracetamol prescribed by her general practitioner.

Reflective questions

You are the registered nurse looking after Beryl and, during a visit, her daughter asks you about her mother's increasing pain levels and what can be done to keep her more comfortable.

› Using the ROPES Model above conduct an interview with Beryl about the causes of her pain and how she would like this managed. What questions would you ask Beryl?

› What impact might her life biography have on her experience of pain?

› What valid pain assessment tool would you use to assess Beryl?

› How often would you redo this assessment?

› What pharmacological and non-pharmacological strategies do you think would be appropriate for Beryl?

Reflective activity

Reflect on an older person you have cared for who has died.
- Did their death match with what we have discussed as a 'good death'?
- If not, what was missing and what steps would you take in the future to address these?
- Did the person you were caring for have pain as a symptom? If 'yes' did they have adequate pain assessments and management?

Summary

- What constitutes a 'good death' for older people may differ and it is important to understand the person's views and wishes.
- Impeccable pain assessment is one of the key elements of providing palliative care and the use of valid and reliable tools is best practice.
- It is important to understand how a person's strengths can impact on the management of pain for people.

Conclusion

A good death requires health professionals to be aware of the individual wishes of the person and their family. Awareness of factors that have been identified by older people as well as health professionals on what constitutes a good death can guide your practice and build upon the strengths of the person. A key feature of a good death is to have as pain free a death as possible. To achieve this good pain assessment and a clear management plan are required.

Further reading

You may like to take a look at the following reading recommendation: Caresearch at http://www.caresearch.com.au

References

Abbey, J., Piller, N., Bellis, A., Esterman, A., Parker, D., Giles, L. & Lowcay, B. (2004). The Abbey Pain Scale: A 1 minute numerical indicator for people with end stage dementia. *International Journal of Palliative Nursing*, 10, 6–13.

Australian Pain Society. (2005). *Pain in Residential Care Facilities: Management Strategies*. North Sydney. Retrieved from http://www.apsoc.org.au/owner/files/9e2c2n.pdf

Blyth, F., March, L., Brnabic, A., Jorm, L., Williamson, M. & Cousin, M. (2001). Chronic pain in Australia: A prevalence study. *Pain*, 127–34.

Field, M. & Cassel, C. (1997). Approaching Death: Improving Care at the End of Life. Washington, DC: National Academy Press.

Fox, P., Raina, P. & Jada, A. (1999). Prevalence and treatment of pain in older adults in nursing homes and other long term care institutions: A systematic review. *Canadian Medical Association Journal*, 160(3), 329–33.

Graybeal, C. (2001). Strengths-based social work assessment: Transforming the dominant paradigm. *Families in Society*, 82(3), 233–43.

Helme, R. & Gibson, S. (1999). Pain in older people. In P. Crombie, S. Linton, L. LeResche & M. Von Korff (Eds.), *Epidemiology of Pain*, 103–12. Seattle: IASP Press.

Herr, K., Bjoro, K. & Decker, S. (2006). Tools for assessment of pain in nonverbal older adults with dementia: A state-of-the-science review. *Journal of Pain and Symptom Management*, 31(2), 170–92.

Herr, K. & Garand, L. (2001). Assessment and measurement of pain in older adults. *Clinical Geriatric Medicine*, 17(3), 457-vi.

Lloyd-Williams, M., Kennedy, V., Sixsmith, A. & Sixsmith, J. (2007). The end of life: A qualitative study of the perceptions of people over the age of 80 on issues surrounding death and dying. *Journal of Pain and Symptom Management*, 34(1), 60–6.

McAuliffe, L., Nay, R., O'Donnell, M. & Fetherstonhaugh, D. (2009). Pain assessment in older people with dementia: Literature review. *Journal of Advanced Nursing*, 65 (1), 2–10. doi: JAN4861 [pii]10.1111/j.1365–2648.2008.04861.x

Smith, R. (2000). A good death. *BMJ*, 320, 129–30.

Steinhauser, K., Clipp, E., McNeilly, M., Christakos, N., McINtyre, L. & Tulsky, J. (2000). In search of a good death: Observations of patients, families and providers. *Annals of Internal Medicine*, 132, 825–32.

Therapeutic Guidelines. (2010). *Palliative Care Version 3, 2010*. Melbourne.

Turk, D. & Melzack, R. (1992). The measurement of pain and the assessment of people experiencing pain. In M. Turk & R. Melzack (Eds.), *Handbook of Pain Assessment* (pp. 3–12). New York: Guildford Press.

Warden, V., Hurley, A. & Volicer, L. (2003). Development and psychometric evaluation of the Pain Assessment in Advanced Dementia (PAINAD) Scale. *Journal of American Directors Association*, 4, 9–15.

World Health Organization. (2014). WHO definition of palliative care. [Search for 'definition of palliative care']. Retrieved from http://www.who.int/cancer/palliative/definition/en/

Glossary

Acute care settings Settings that provide short-term medical treatment, usually in a hospital, for patients having an acute illness or injury or recovering from surgery.

Acute on chronic pain Pain that is between acute and chronic, and may also be known as subacute pain.

Acute pain The body's normal response to damage such as a cut, an infection or other physical injuries. This type of pain usually comes on fast and often goes away in no more than a few weeks or months if treated properly.

Advance care directive A legal document that sets out instructions that consent to or refuse specified medical treatments. It is designed to be enacted when the person is no longer able to make informed decisions.

Advance care planning A process whereby a person's values, beliefs and preferences are made known so that they can be used to guide decision making in circumstances where the person is no longer able to do so.

Aged Care Funding Instrument appraisal Used for determining the level of care payments for residents in residential aged care facilities.

Aged care system Provides the framework for older people to have timely access to appropriate care and support services.

Ageing demographics Statistical data relating to the ageing population and particular cohorts within it.

Ageism A set of beliefs, attitudes, norms and values used to justify age-based prejudice and discrimination.

Alzheimer's disease The most common type of dementia.

Anti-psychotic medication A class of medication that is used to treat psychosis, as well as mental and emotional conditions.

Anxiety disorder A medical condition in which the individual suffers from persistent and excessive worry.

Behavioural and psychological symptoms of dementia Distressing and non-cognitive symptoms of dementia such as agitation and aggression.

Capabilities Model of Dementia Care A model of dementia care informed by the capabilities approach.

Case management An essential aspect of care delivery provided to individuals and including ongoing monitoring of support, detailed planning of clinical care and other aspects of delivery. Increases in intensity as need of clients becomes more complex.

Chronic disease A disease that is persistent or otherwise long-lasting in its effects. The term 'chronic' is usually applied when the course of the disease lasts for more than three months.

Chronic pain Pain that has lasted longer than three to six months and does not resolve in response to treatment.

Client advocate Someone who advances the rights of older persons and educates others regarding negative stereotypes of ageing.

Clinical decision making A balance of experience, awareness, knowledge and information gathering, using appropriate assessment tools, colleagues and evidence-based practice as guidance.

Cochrane Collaboration An independent non-profit organisation consisting of a group of more than 31 000 volunteers in more than 120 countries. The collaboration was formed to organise medical research information in a systematic way in the interests of evidence-based medicine.

Cognitive behavioural therapy An individualised approach that helps the individual to learn or relearn healthier skills and habits and to reduce negative thoughts.

Co-morbidity factors Factors that increase risk of developing chronic disease, such as depression.

Complexity Focus on multiple spheres of physical, functional, psychological and social care.

Consumer directed care Described as both a philosophy and an orientation to a service delivery option where consumers control and choose the services they get, including what, when, how, where and who provides those services.

Culturally competent Responding effectively to cultural and linguistic needs of clients and caregivers.

Cultural safety The client rather than the nurse or health practitioner defines if the care is safe.

Curative Health care traditionally oriented towards seeking a cure for an existent disease or medical condition.

Delirium An acute confused state lasting from hours to a few weeks.

Dementia An umbrella term used to describe a collection of symptoms caused by disorders affecting the brain.

Depression A state of low mood that has serious implications for physical and mental health.

E-health A system that enables a personally controlled, secure online summary of a client's health information.

Electroconvulsive therapy A procedure that involves the passing of electric currents through the brain to trigger a seizure.

End of life care Care in the last days or week of life.

End of life care pathway A structured document that focuses on care required in the last few days or week of life.

Endorsed enrolled nurses Second level nurses who provide nursing care, working under the direction and supervision of registered nurses. Have endorsement to administer medications.

Epidemiology The study of health amongst populations.

Euthanasia The act of deliberately ending the life of a patient for the purpose of ending intolerable pain and/or suffering.

Evidence-based practice The practice of health care in which the practitioner systematically finds, appraises and uses the most current and valid research findings as the basis for clinical decisions.

Family caregiver An unpaid caregiver (family, friend or neighbour) who provides care, in a voluntary capacity, for another's physical, emotional and developmental well-being.

Family Involvement in Care (FIC) intervention Derived from evidence that working partnerships based on knowledge exchange and negotiation of roles can improve well-being for staff, families and people with dementia.

Frailty 'A state of vulnerability to poor resolution of homeostasis after a stressor event and it is a consequence of cumulative decline in many physiological systems' (Clegg et al., 2013, p. 752).

Functional assessment Comprehensive evaluation of physical and cognitive abilities required to maintain independence.

Functional incontinence Occurs as a result of impairment stopping the person getting to the toilet on time.

Geriatric The clinical practice of medicine that encompasses the gerontology, pathology and complexities of ageing.

Geriatric Anxiety Inventory A 20-item self-report or interviewer administered scale that measures anxiety in older people.

Geriatric Depression Scale A well validated scale that assists in screening older people for depression.

Geriatric syndrome Occurs when the unique features of common health conditions in the elderly, such as delirium, falls, incontinence and frailty, are highly prevalent, multifactorial, and associated with substantial morbidity and poor outcomes.

Gerontology The study of ageing.

Gold Standards Framework A model of palliative care used in the UK across a range of settings including long-term care.

Guided imagery A program of directed thoughts and suggestions that guide a person towards a relaxed state.

Health The ability of older adults to function at their highest capacity despite the presence of age related changes and risk factors.

Health promotion interventions Interventions that focus on behaviour changes, including disease prevention and health maintenance.

High care People who require almost complete assistance with most daily living activities as well as accommodation, meals, laundry and room cleaning.

Holistic care A system of comprehensive patient care that considers the physical, emotional, social, economic and spiritual needs of the person; his or her response to illness; and the effect of the illness on the ability to meet self-care needs.

Hospice Physical building where care is provided (Australia); physical building and philosophy (New Zealand).

Human lifespan How long a member of the human species can potentially live.

Incidence Risk associated with disease.

Informal care Regular, sustained care to a person in need of support on an unpaid basis.

Interdisciplinary Involving the scope of two or more distinct disciplines.

Intradisciplinary Occurring within the scope of a discipline, between people active in the discipline.

King's Model A nursing model of care that focuses on the importance of interaction.

Life expectancy The number of years that an individual is expected to live as determined by statistics.

Life limiting illness An illness in which it is expected that death will be a direct consequence.

Lifespan The period between birth and death.

Local hospital networks Small groups of local hospitals, or an individual hospital, linking services within a region or through specialist networks across a state or territory.

Long-term care settings Residential care for individuals above the age of 65 or with a chronic or disabling condition that needs constant supervision.

Low care People who require accommodation, meals, laundry, room cleaning as well as help with personal care and possibly nursing care.

Magnetic field therapy Involves the placing of magnetic devices on or near the body to relieve pain.

Major depression A depression that is not biological and is likely to be related to psychological causes such as stressful life events.

Medicare Local Program Primary health care practices that coordinate and deliver services based on community need, including after-hours GP services, immunisation, mental health support, targeted and tailored services for those in need, and e-health.

Melancholic depression A severe biological form of depression in which the person experiences low energy, poor concentration, and slowed or agitated movements.

Mixed incontinence A mixture of different types of incontinence.

Morbidity Increasing risk of exposure to disease.

Mortality The measure of the risk of disease severity.

Multidisciplinary Combining or involving several academic disciplines or professional specialisations in an approach to a topic or problem.

Multidisciplinary team Composed of members from more than one discipline so that the team can offer a greater breadth of services to patients.

Namaste Care™ A program of person-centred care for people with dementia.

Neuropathic pain This is caused by damage to nerves.

Neuroticism A long-term tendency to be in a negative state.

Nociceptive pain This is caused by stimulation of nerve endings in skin and deep tissue.

Nursing Interventions Classification A comprehensive, research-based, standardised classification of interventions that nurses perform.

Nursing models The frameworks on which nursing care can focus.

Old-old People aged 85 years and above.

Orem's Model A nursing model of care that focuses on the concept of self-care and integrates the theory of human needs.

Overflow incontinence Result of an inability to fully empty the bladder, resulting in frequent small volumes of urine being released.

Palliative approach The goal is to improve the person's level of comfort and function, and address physical, psychological, spiritual and social needs.

Palliative Approach Toolkit An evidence-based resource for providing a palliative approach in residential aged care facilities.

Palliative care A philosophy of care.

Palliative care case conferences Multidisciplinary meetings with the resident, family, general practitioner and nursing care team. The focus is on palliative and end of life care.

Palliative care clinical nurse consultants Registered nurses with specialist knowledge in palliative care.

Paradigm A world view underlying the development of theories and models.

Partnership models Derive from the view that families themselves are clients and a potential resource for improving quality of care for the resident with dementia.

Person-centred care Treatment and care provided by health services that places the person at the centre of their own care and considers the needs of the older person's carers.

Personhood The standing or status bestowed on a human being.

Philosophy The values and beliefs of a discipline

Population ageing Refers to an increase in the proportion of older people accompanied by a reduction in the proportion of children, alongside a reduction in the proportion of people of working age.

Prevalence Percentage of the population affected by a disease or condition.

Primary care First point of health care delivered in, and to, people living in their communities.

Primary nursing care Comprehensive, individualised care performed by the same nurse.

Prognosis Includes the expected duration, function and a description of the course of the disease.

Psycho-education Education to help with the psychological stress of a condition such as pain.

Quality of life An individual's perception of their position in life in the context of the culture and value systems in which they live and in relation to their goals, expectations, standards and concerns.

Randomised controlled trials Used to test the efficacy and effectiveness of interventions and involve participants being allocated at random to receive several interventions, including a comparison or control.

Rating Anxiety in Dementia (RAID) scale A valid and reliable scale for measuring anxiety in people with dementia.

Rehabilitation A treatment or treatments designed to facilitate the process of recovery from injury, illness or disease to as normal a condition as possible.

Relational approach Refers to the importance of relationships in providing care.

Relationship-centred care Centres on the importance of relationships.

Risk factor(s) Behaviour(s) that increase risk of disease.

Schizophrenia A mental disorder that is characterised by a breakdown in thinking and poor emotional responses.

Science A unified body of knowledge about phenomena that is based on agreed-upon evidence.

Screening and proactive assessments Detect problems and identify potential for multi-dimensional health or functional impairment at an early stage in order to initiate interventions designed to improve health, for example, diabetes, depression.

Self-efficacy The ability of the person to regulate their motivation, thought processes and emotional states, and appropriate behavioural changes. Self-efficacy affects the older person's functional status during rehabilitation.

Senescence Physiological progressive deterioration of body systems that can increase mortality risk in an older person.

Senses Framework A framework that focuses on six senses.

Snoezelen A multi-sensorial stimulation of the primary senses, i.e. hearing, touch, taste, smell and sight, through stimulants such as essential oils and music.

Social capital Reflects an individual's relationships and their standing in their social community.

Specialist palliative care Involves referral to a specialised palliative care team or health practitioner.

Strengths-based care An approach to care that focuses on individuals' strengths rather than pathologies.

Stress incontinence The loss of urine when pressure is exerted on the bladder.

Subacute care Provides assessment and rehabilitation for complex conditions following or preceding acute care admission. Usually for a maximum of three months.

Subacute extended care unit Distinct unit located within an acute care general hospital that utilises licensed long-term care beds.

Substitute decision maker Someone who acts on behalf of a person who lacks capacity.

Suicide The act of intentionally causing one's own death.

Syndrome A group of signs and symptoms that occur together and characterise a particular condition.

Team nursing Involves the use of a team leader and team members who deliver care to a group of patients.

Theory The search for an explanation.

Total incontinence Uncontrollable leaking of urine.

Transition Care Programs Programs for older people who have been in hospital, but need more help to recover and time to make a decision about the best place for them to live in the longer term.

Urge incontinence Sudden, intense urge to urinate, followed by an involuntary loss of urine.

Urinary incontinence An inability to control the flow of urine that results in involuntary urination.

VIPS The four main concepts of person-centred care.

Wellness Outcome (or positive functional consequence) for older adults whose well-being and quality of life is improved through nursing interventions.

Young onset dementia This refers to people with onset of dementia before 65 years of age.

Index

Printed in the United States
by Bookmasters

Printed in the United States
By Bookmasters